LASER SURGERY IN OPHTHALMOLOGY
Practical Applications

LASER SURGERY IN OPHTHALMOLOGY
Practical Applications

Edited by

Thomas A. Weingeist, MD, PhD
Professor and Head
Department of Ophthalmology
University of Iowa College of Medicine
University of Iowa Hospitals and Clinics
Iowa City, Iowa

Scott R. Sneed, MD
Assistant Professor
Department of Ophthalmology
W. K. Kellogg Eye Center
The University of Michigan
Ann Arbor, Michigan

Foreword by
J. Donald M. Gass, MD
Professor of Ophthalmology
Bascom Palmer Eye Institute
University of Miami School of Medicine
Miami, Florida

APPLETON & LANGE
Norwalk, Connecticut/San Mateo, California

0-8385-7903-5

Copyright © 1992 by Appleton & Lange
A Publishing Division of Prentice Hall

92 93 94 95 96 / 10 9 8 7 6 5 4 3 2 1

Prentice Hall International (UK) Limited, *London*
Prentice Hall of Australia Pty. Limited, *Sydney*
Prentice Hall Canada, Inc., *Toronto*
Prentice Hall Hispanoamericana, S.A., *Mexico*
Prentice Hall of India Private Limited, *New Delhi*
Prentice Hall of Japan, Inc., *Tokyo*
Simon & Schuster Asia Pte. Ltd., *Singapore*
Editora Prentice-Hall do Brasil, Ltda., *Rio de Janeiro*
Prentice Hall, *Englewood Cliffs, New Jersey*

Library of Congress Cataloging-in-Publication Data

Laser surgery in ophthalmology: practical applications / edited by
  Thomas A. Weingeist, Scott R. Sneed.
    p. cm.
  ISBN 0-8385-7903-5
  1. Lasers in ophthalmology. 2. Eye—Surgery. I. Weingeist,
  Thomas A. II. Sneed, Scott R.
  [DNLM: 1. Eye Diseases—surgery. 2. Laser Surgery—methods. WW
  168 P895]
RE86.P73 1992
617.7'1—dc20
DNLM/DLC
for Library of Congress   91-22411
                                                              CIP

Acquisitions Editor: Joan Meyer
Production Editor: Eileen Lagoss Burns
Designer: Janice Barsevich

PRINTED IN THE UNITED STATES OF AMERICA

This volume is dedicated to our fathers
Samson Weingeist, MD
and
Robert J. Sneed, MD
teacher, friend, and ophthalmologist

Contents

Preface

The concept of this book initially arose from a course on laser photocoagulation given at the University of Iowa in 1982. Since that time, many technological improvements have been developed for treating ocular disease with laser surgery. Similarly, results of numerous controlled clinical trials (Diabetic Retinopathy Study, Macular Photocoagulation Study, Early Treatment Diabetic Retinopathy Study, Branch Retinal Vein Occlusion Study) have proven the efficacy of laser surgery in the treatment of ocular disease as outlined in NIH Publication No. 90-2910 entitled *Clinical Trials Supported by the National Eye Institute.*

The aim of this book is to clearly describe laser techniques for more common and some infrequently encountered ocular diseases. The techniques of laser surgery described in this book have been successfully used by many ophthalmic surgeons, but are not necessarily the only ways in which the ophthalmologist might treat a particular disease entity. Variations of the techniques described herein are successfully used by ophthalmologists.

This book is intended for ophthalmology residents, fellows, and for general ophthalmologists who may use laser in treating more common ocular disease. Ophthalmology subspecialists may find the book useful as a reference when treating less common ocular disorders. Laser surgeons should find the tables describing laser parameters and goals for specific ocular diseases to be particularly helpful in planning and performing laser surgery. Variations of the described techniques may develop based upon clinical experience and further advances in the ophthalmic literature. This book is not intended as a "how to" text for ophthalmologists not trained in laser surgery. Formal "hands on" laser surgery under the direct supervision of an experienced laser surgeon is necessary for learning the techniques of laser surgery.

Several aspects of laser surgery in ophthalmology are not covered in this text. Use of the CO_2, the Argon laser, and the scalpel Nd:YAG lasers in oculoplastic surgery is becoming increasingly popular in treating orbital and ocular plastic conditions. Similarly, the excimer laser is being used in keratorefractive surgery and may become a more practical tool as more clinical results are published. The diode laser has been successfully used to treat various retinal diseases, and to perform laser peripheral iridectomies and cyclodestruction. The small size and low maintenance of the unit as well as the good penetration of retinal edema and cataractous lenses are advantages that may lead to more widespread use of the diode laser. The ability to "choose" a particular wavelength makes the dye laser an attractive instrument for the laser surgeon. The dye yellow wavelength is highly absorbed by hemoglobin and may be useful for treating vascular lesions of the eye. Increased use of these "newer" lasers may develop as more laboratory and clinical experience is acquired.

This book is the product of a combined effort of many people, particularly the contributing authors and their staff. Our wives, Catherine and Cristy, and our children shared in their own ways, the burden of producing this book. The editors are particularly grateful to Ramona Weber who helped to organize the materials for this project and assiduously typed multiple revisions of the manuscript. We would also like to extend our thanks and appreciation to Joan Meyer, Medical Editor of Appleton & Lange, and her staff for their patience and support throughout the creation and production of this book.

Thomas A. Weingeist, MD, PhD
Scott R. Sneed, MD

Contributors

Wallace L.M. Alward, MD
Assistant Professor
Director Glaucoma Service
Department of Ophthalmology
University of Iowa College of Medicine
University of Iowa Hospitals and Clinics
Iowa City, Iowa

Christopher F. Blodi, MD
Associate Professor
Associate Director of Vitreoretinal Service
Department of Ophthalmology
University of Iowa College of Medicine
University of Iowa Hospitals and Clinics
Iowa City, Iowa

George H. Bresnick
Professor and Acting Chairman
Department of Ophthalmology
University of Wisconsin-Madison
Madison, Wisconsin

Patrick J. Caskey, MD
North Bay Vitreoretinal Consultants
Santa Rosa, California

Consultant, Retina Service
Pacific Presbyterian Medical Center
San Francisco, California

Assistant Clinical Professor
University of California
San Francisco, California

Patrick Coonan, MD
North Bay Vitreoretinal Consultants
Santa Rosa, California

Consultant, Retina Service
Pacific Presbyterian Medical Center
San Francisco, California

Assistant Clinical Professor
University of California
San Francisco, California

Matthew D. Davis, MD
Professor
Department of Ophthalmology
University of Wisconsin-Madison
Madison, Wisconsin

James C. Folk, MD
Professor
Director of Vitreoretinal Service
Department of Ophthalmology
University of Iowa College of Medicine
University of Iowa Hospitals and Clinics
Iowa City, Iowa

Vernon M. Hermsen, MD
Bellville, Illinois

Karen M. Joos, MD, PhD
Resident
Department of Ophthalmology
University of Iowa College of Medicine
University of Iowa Hospitals and Clinics
Iowa City, Iowa

Alan E. Kimura, MD
Assistant Professor
Director Electrodiagnostic Laboratory
Department of Ophthalmology
University of Iowa College of Medicine
University of Iowa Hospitals and Clinics
Iowa City, Iowa

Deen G. King, MD
Assistant Clinical Professor
University of South Florida
College of Medicine
Tampa, Florida

Hansjoerg E. Kolder, MD
Professor
Director Cataract Service

Department of Ophthalmology
University of Iowa College of Medicine
University of Iowa Hospitals and Clinics
Iowa City, Iowa

Peter Reed Pavan, MD
Associate Professor
Director Vitreoretinal Service
University of South Florida
College of Medicine
Tampa, Florida

Jose S. Pulido, MD
Assistant Professor
Department of Ophthalmology
University of Iowa College of Medicine
University of Iowa Hospitals and Clinics
Iowa City, Iowa

Michael B. Rivers, MD
Vitreoretinal Fellow
Department of Ophthalmology
University of Iowa College of Medicine
University of Iowa Hospitals and Clinics
Iowa City, Iowa

E. George Rosanelli, MD
Assistant Clinical Professor
University of South Florida
College of Medicine
Tampa, Florida

Stephen R. Russell, MD
Assistant Professor
Director Vitreoretinal Service
Bethesda Eye Institute
St. Louis University Medical Center
St. Louis, Missouri

Scott R. Sneed, MD
Assistant Professor
Department of Ophthalmology
W.K. Kellogg Eye Center
The University of Michigan
Ann Arbor, Michigan

Warren M. Sobol, M.D.
Vitreoretinal Fellow
Department of Ophthalmology
University of Iowa College of Medicine
University of Iowa Hospitals and Clinics
Iowa City, Iowa

Ingolf Wallow, MD
Professor
Department of Ophthalmology
University of Wisconsin-Madison
Madison, Wisconsin

Robert C. Watzke, MD
Professor
Director Retina Service
University Ophthalmic Consultants
The Oregon Health Sciences University
Portland, Oregon

Thomas A. Weingeist, MD, PhD
Professor and Head
Department of Ophthalmology
University of Iowa College of Medicine
University of Iowa Hospitals and Clinics
Iowa City, Iowa

Mitchell D. Wolf, MD
Fellow Associate
Department of Ophthalmology
University of Iowa College of Medicine
University of Iowa Hospitals and Clinics
Iowa City, Iowa

Foreword

In 1949, Meyer-Schwickerath introduced ophthalmology to xenon photocoagulation, and ophthalmology subsequently introduced laser photocoagulation to the medical world. During the past decade, the rapid acceleration of laser technology has extended into almost every subspecialty of medicine. What began as a tool used by a few ophthalmologists for the treatment of several diseases of the ocular fundus has expanded to the treatment of disorders affecting virtually every part of the eye and adnexal structures. Laser photocoagulation is rapidly becoming part of the therapeutic armamentarium of every ophthalmologist. While controlled clinical trials have provided guidelines or indications and techniques for photocoagulation treatment of some of the more common ocular disorders, less information is available concerning management of other diseases. This very readable book will be helpful to those experienced, as well as those less experienced, in improving their clinical judgment and skills in the techniques of photocoagulation. Although not designed as a primer for those with no training in photocoagulation, it includes informative introductory chapters that review the anatomy of the eye, principles of photocoagulation, and the histopathologic changes induced by laser.

The primary contribution of this book is the presentation by a number of seasoned and skilled practitioners of their experience in photocoagulation treatment of a wide variety of ocular diseases. Included are individual nuances of thought and technique that will be helpful to even the most experienced in photocoagulation. The authors have succeeded in making this a practical guide for the laser surgeon.

J. Donald M. Gass, MD

CHAPTER 1

Anatomy of the Eye

Thomas A. Weingeist

- **The Chamber Angle**
- **The Iris**
- **The Retina**
- **The Choroid**
- **References**

Success in laser surgery is dependent in part on a clear understanding of the anatomy of the eye. Knowledge of the location and the type of ocular pigments also is essential. The most important pigments are melanin, hemoglobin, and xanthophyll. The transparency of the ocular media allows radiant energy to enter the interior of the eye without appreciable loss. Coagulation of the eye tissues is due in large part to absorption of electromagnetic radiation by pigments and conversion of this energy into heat.

The main purpose of this chapter is to review those parts of the ocular anatomy that are important in laser photocoagulation therapy. Attention to anatomic details can mean the difference between success and failure. The anatomy of the following structures is reviewed: the anterior chamber angle, the iris, the retina, and the choroid.[1–3]

THE CHAMBER ANGLE

The chamber angle, which lies at the juncture of the cornea and the iris, consists of (1) Schwalbe's line, (2) the trabecular meshwork and canal of Schlemm, (3) the scleral spur, (4) the anterior border of the ciliary body, and (5) the iris (Fig. 1–1).

Many of the chamber angle structures can be visualized by gonioscopy. Schwalbe's line, the termination of Descemet's membrane, often can be seen as a hazy zone at the border of the cornea. If a thin slit beam is used to illuminate the angle obliquely, a corneal wedge is formed by the two converging beams at Schwalbe's line, which is located at the anterior border of the trabecular meshwork. Iris processes frequently can be seen extending from the surface of the iris into the trabecular meshwork. They should not be confused with peripheral anterior synechiae. The ciliary body is visible above the iris root. The longitudinal muscle fibers of the ciliary body insert into the trabec-

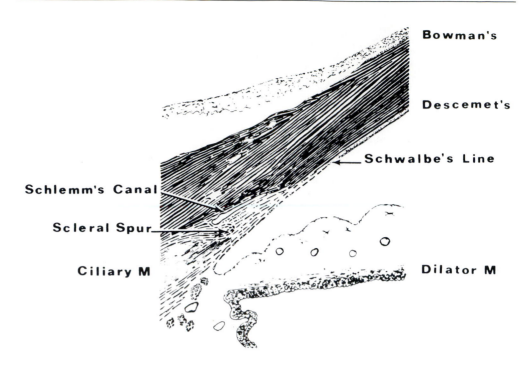

Figure 1–1. Schematic diagram of anterior chamber angle and iris.

ular meshwork. The scleral spur is formed by collagen fibers that invaginate between the anterior portion of the ciliary body and the canal of Schlemm. Schlemm's canal lies in the scleral sulcus just anterior to the scleral spur, between the middle and the posterior third of the trabecular meshwork. It appears as a faint gray line, or if blood has refluxed from the episcleral veins via the collector channels, it will stand out as a fine red line.

The pigmentation of the trabecular meshwork is variable. It tends to be greater in individuals with brown irises than in those with blue irises. However, the only reliable means of determining the degree of pigmentation is by gonioscopy. The lower chamber angle often is more pigmented than the upper. The melanin granules located in the trabecular beams are structurally identical to those found in the posterior pigmented layer of the iris.

The trabecular meshwork consists of a series of thin, perforated connective tissue sheets arranged in a laminar pattern. Each sheet is comprised of several components: a central core of collagen and elastic fibrils surrounded by a thin basal lamina and a single continuous row of thin endothelial cells with multiple pinocytotic vesicles. Intertrabecular and transtrabecular spaces exist throughout the meshwork.

The canal of Schlemm closely resembles the structure of a large lymphatic. It is formed by a continuous layer of nonfenestrated endothelial cells and a thin connective tissue wall. Tight junctions join the lateral walls of the endothelial cells. Collector channels arising from Schlemm's canal drain through a circuitous route into the aqueous veins.

THE IRIS

The iris is the most anterior extension of the uveal tract. It is comprised of blood vessels and connective tissue, in addition to melanocytes and pigmented cells, which are responsible for its distinctive color. The iris is unusual, since it fails to undergo wound repair even if its cut edges are sutured together.

The anterior surface of the iris normally is avascular, and it is not covered by a continuous layer of cells. The aqueous humor flows freely through the loose stroma, which contains melanocytes, collagen fibrils, blood vessels, and nerves.

The posterior border of the iris can be divided into two layers. The anterior layer comprises the dilator muscle. The posterior layer forms the pigmented layer of the iris. Ectropion uveae with and without rubeosis iridis occurs when these two neuroectodermal layers curve around the pupillary margin and extend onto the anterior surface of the iris. In order for surgical or laser iridotomy to succeed, an opening must exist through both pigmented layers of the iris.

THE RETINA

The retina is a thin, transparent structure that differentiates from the inner and the outer layers of the optic cup. The structure of the outer, pigmented epithelial layer is relatively simple compared with the overlying inner or neurosensory retina (Fig. 1–2).

The retinal pigment epithelium (RPE) consists of hexagon-shaped cells that extend from the optic disc posteriorly to the ora serrata anteriorly. The pigmented granules within the cytoplasm are primarily responsible for the absorption of radiant energy that occurs during laser photocoagulation.

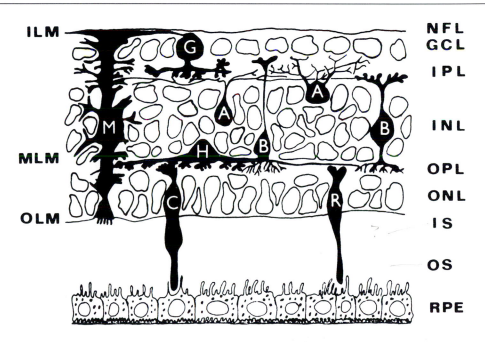

Figure 1–2. Cross-sectional representation of retinal architecture. ILM, inner limiting membrane; MLM, middle limiting membrane; OLM, outer limiting membrane; NFL, nerve fiber layer; GCL, ganglion cell layer; IPL, inner plexiform layer; INL, inner nuclear layer; OPL, outer plexiform layer; IS, inner segments; OS, outer segments; RPE, retinal pigment epithelium; ONL, outer nuclear layer. A, amacrine cell; B, bipolar cell; C, cone photoreceptor cell; G, ganglion cell; H, horizontal cell; M, Müller cell; R, rod photoreceptor cell. *(Modified from Dowling JR: Organization of vertebrate retinas.* Invest Ophthalmol. *1970;9:655–680.)*

Destruction of the RPE by laser photocoagulation is repaired through a combination of migration of adjacent RPE cells and invasion of tissue macrophages. Adult RPE cells seldom undergo mitosis.

Important regional differences exist in the structure of the RPE. Cells in the fovea are taller and thinner and contain more and larger melanosomes. This accounts in part for the decreased transmission of choroidal fluorescence observed during fundus fluorescein angiography. RPE cells in the peripheral fundus are broader, lower, and less pigmented.

The inner retina consists of neural, glial, and vascular cells. Because the neurosensory retina is essentially transparent, it is affected by laser photocoagulation only indirectly. Conversion of radiant energy into heat occurs as a result of light absorption by pigment granules in the RPE, by hemoglobin in the vascular system, and by xanthophyll in the inner layers of the macula.

Important structural and functional differences also exist within the retina. The retina varies greatly in cross-sectional thickness. It is thinnest in the foveola and in the ora serrata (0.1 mm) and thickest in the papillomacular bundle (0.23 mm) temporal to the optic disc. The overlying nerve fibers in the region of the papillomacular bundle can be spared if the proper parameters are used and judicious care is taken in administering laser therapy in this area.

The inner portion of the retina is supplied by branches of the central retinal artery. One or more cilioretinal arteries are present in 30 percent of eyes.[4] The blood vessels in the retina, like those in the central nervous system, contain tight junctions that help to maintain the blood–retinal barrier. Only near the disc do the retinal venules and arterioles contain smooth muscle cells. Elsewhere, they consist of nonfenestrated endothelial cells and intramural cells or pericytes that share a common basement membrane. None of the retinal blood vessels possess elastic fibers as in the choroid or elsewhere in the body.

The foveal avascular zone (FAZ) has become an important landmark for the treatment of subretinal neovascular membranes. However, its appearance in fundus fluorescein angiograms is highly variable. The diameter of the FAZ varies from 250 μm to more than 600 μm, and in many instances, a truly avascular zone cannot be identified (Fig. 1–3).[5]

The width of the superior and the inferior temporal veins is approximately 125 μm near the disc margin. Either vessel can, therefore, serve as an internal marker in judging small distances in the posterior pole.

A great deal of confusion still exists among both clinicians and anatomists regarding the terms macula lutea, macula, posterior pole, fovea, and foveola.

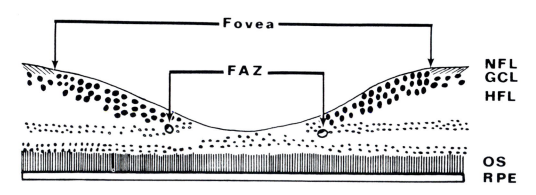

Figure 1–3. Schematic diagram of macula. FAZ, foveal avascular zone; NFL, nerve fiber layer; GCL, ganglion cell layer; HFL, Henle fiber layer; OS, outer segments; RPE, retinal pigment epithelium. *(From Am Acad Ophthalmol, Basic and Clinical Science Course. Section I: Fundamentals of Ophthalmology; 1990–1991, p. 73.)*

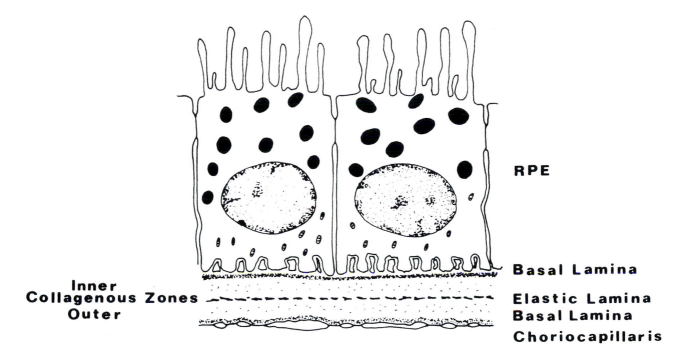

Inner
Collagenous Zones
Outer

RPE

Basal Lamina

Elastic Lamina
Basal Lamina

Choriocapillaris

Figure 1–4. Schematic diagram of retinal pigment epithelium and Bruch's membrane. RPE, retinal pigment epithelium. *(From Am Acad Ophthalmol. Basic and Clinical Science Course. Section I: Fundamentals of Ophthalmology; 1990–1991, p. 83.)*

There is a tendency among retina specialists to regard the *macula* as the area within the temporal vascular arcades. Histologically, it is the region where more than one layer of ganglion cell nuclei can be found.[6,7]

The posterior pole encompasses the macula and optic disk in addition to a zone 1-2 disc diameters anteriorly.

The term *macula lutea*, which means yellow spot, is based on the appearance of the central retina in dissected cadaver eyes. Neither the chemical composition nor the location of the yellow pigment is completely understood. The pigment is probably a xanthophyll. Lipofuscin granules, which are known to be yellowish in color, have been observed by electron microscopy in the cytoplasm of ganglion cells in the perifoveal region.

The *foveola* is a central depression within the fovea. Its center is located about 3.5 mm temporal and 0.8 mm inferior to the center of the optic disc. It is approximately 350 μm in diameter and 0.1 mm in thickness. The floor or base of the fovea sometimes is referred to as the "umbo." Clinically, the borders of the foveola merge imperceptibly with the fovea.

The *fovea* is about 1.5 mm in diameter, or about the size of the surface of the optic nerve head. Clinically, its borders are inexact. In children and young adults, it is sometimes evident ophthalmoscopically as an oval light reflex.

THE CHOROID

Bruch's membrane appears by light microscopy as a PAS positive membrane, but in fact it is not a true membrane. Five distinct layers have been defined by electron microscopy. They are from within out: (1) the inner basal lamina of the RPE, (2) the inner collagenous zone, (3) the central, porous band of elastic fibers, (4) the outer collagenous zone, and (5) the basal lamina of the outer layer of the choriocapillaris. Bruch's membrane is highly permeable and undergoes characteristic aging changes and alterations from disease processes, which make it prone to neovascular infiltration from the choriocapillaris (Fig. 1–4).

The choriocapillaris is structurally a continuous layer of capillaries lying in a single plane beneath the RPE. The vessel walls are extremely thin, contain multiple fenestrations, and lack tight junctions, such as those found in retinal vessels. As a result, they are highly permeable and leak fluorescein as well as other small molecules.

The choroid beneath the choriocapillaris contains a middle and outer layer of large, nonfenestrated vessels. Penetrating laser photocoagulation may damage these vessels, since large numbers of pigmented melanocytes are located adjacent to them in the uveal stroma.

REFERENCES

1. Fine BS, Yanoff M: *Ocular Histology, A Text and Atlas*, 2nd ed. Hagerstown, MD: Harper & Row; 1979:359.
2. Hogan MJ, Alvarado JA, Weddell JE: *Histology of the Human Eye, An Atlas and Textbook*. Philadelphia: WB Saunders Co; 1971:687.
3. Basic and Clinical Science Course Section 1. *Fundamentals and Principles of Ophthalmology*. San Francisco: American Academy of Ophthalmology; 1989–1990:53–86.
4. Justice J, Lehmann RP: Cilioretinal arteries—a study based on review of stereo fundus photographs and fluorescein angiographic findings. *Arch Ophthalmol* 1976; 94:1355–1358.
5. Bird AC, Weale RA: On the retinal vasculature of the human fovea. *Exp Eye Res* 1974;19:409–417.
6. Orth DH, Fine BS, Fagman W, Quirk TC: Clarification of foveomacular nomenclature and grid for quantitation of macular disorders. *Trans Am Acad Ophthalmol Otolaryngol* 1977;83:OP506–514.
7. Spitznas M: Anatomical features of the human macula. In: L'Esperance F, ed. *Current Diagnosis and Management of Choroiretinal Diseases*. St. Louis: CV Mosby; 1977:279–286.

CHAPTER 2

Contact and Noncontact Lenses in Photocoagulation Therapy

Alan E. Kimura

- ■ **Introduction**
- ■ **Purposes of Accessory Lenses**
- ■ **Types of Lens Design**
- ■ **Features Common to Contact Lenses Used for Laser Surgery**
- ■ **Coupling Solutions**
- ■ **Noncontact Lenses for Laser Surgery**
- ■ **Commonly Used Lenses for Anterior Segment Laser Surgery**
- ■ **Commonly Used Lenses for Posterior Segment Laser Surgery**
- ■ **Summary**
- ■ **References**

INTRODUCTION

The purpose of this chapter is to review lenses that are used commonly in ophthalmic photocoagulation therapy. Detailed discussions of optics can be found elsewhere in several excellent sources. Only the practical considerations, such as relative spot size and magnification, are discussed here. Although there are many new styles of lenses on the market today, most of this chapter is devoted to the time-tested lenses that enjoy widespread use.

PURPOSES OF ACCESSORY LENSES

Accessory lenses are required for optimal visualization and treatment of intraocular structures. Basically, an accessory lens is required to image these structures at a point where they can be reimaged by the slit lamp.

Lenses that are coupled to the corneal surface are preferred for both viewing the pathology and safely delivering the energy of the laser. In rare cases, however, the laser may be delivered through a handheld lens that is not against the cornea. A fragile corneal epithelial surface, immature surgical wound, and patient discomfort from recent surgery are relative indications for considering a noncontact type of lens. Laser should be delivered through a slit-lamp system for optimal viewing. Laser delivery through an indirect ophthalmoscopic system and handheld +20 or +28 diopter (D) lens occasionally is useful for demarcating retinal pathology when faced with a subtotal gas fill of the vitreous cavity. The optical disturbances found at the gas–fluid meniscus can be minimized by positioning the patient on the back or side.

TYPES OF LENS DESIGN

Accessory lenses are of two types, noncontact and contact. Examples of noncontact lenses are the Hruby and the +90 D lenses. The contact type lenses include the Goldmann fundus lens, the Goldmann three-mirror lens, and the Rodenstock panfunduscopic lens.

FEATURES COMMON TO CONTACT LENSES USED FOR LASER SURGERY

All contact lenses for laser surgery have a concave posterior surface to fit the corneal curvature, and some have a flange to stabilize the lens and minimize the effects of blinking by the patient. Models with a knurled flange provide the examiner with better control of the lens. The lens elements and mirrors are made of glass and are surrounded by either a polymethyl methacrylate or aluminum shell.[1]

Another important feature is the use of antireflection coatings on the lens surfaces. They not only improve the image quality by decreasing the amount of scattered white light from the biomicroscope but also reduce reflected laser light, which would be backscattered by the anterior surface of the accessory lens.[1] Laser surgery thus is delivered more accurately and safely with lenses using antireflection coatings.

COUPLING SOLUTIONS

Hydroxypropyl methylcellulose (2.0%–2.5%) is used commonly to form a bond between the cornea and the contact lens. This material provides some protection to the corneal epithelium. However, the viscous methylcellulose solutions are difficult to irrigate from the cornea, and their use may create suboptimal photographic documentation after contact lens examination.

Several contact lens solutions have been described that provide excellent postcontact lens examination clarity for subsequent clinical examination or photography. Moffett recently reported using 1.0% carboxymethylcellulose sodium for use as an ophthalmic lubricant. It has a viscosity and adherence greater than saline and, at the same time, provides excellent optical clarity after contact lens removal.[2] Alternatively, Gass described using balanced salt solution for contact lens examination.[3] The balanced salt solution is technically somewhat more difficult to use, and bubbles may form between the cornea and the contact lens unless the lens is placed on the cornea with the patient's head tilted forward and the contact lens in a horizontal position such that the balanced salt solution does not spill out of the contact lens. The balanced salt solution creates excellent corneal adherence and leaves good corneal clarity after contact lens removal.

NONCONTACT LENSES FOR LASER SURGERY

Contact lens use may be a relative contraindication in some patients who require laser surgery (patients with recent surgery or trauma or patients with abnormal corneal epithelium secondary to diabetes mellitus, anterior basement membrane corneal dystrophy, or recurrent corneal erosion). Several publications document the successful use of a +60 D lens and a +90 D lens for retinal photocoagulation.[4-6] Successful use of these lenses has been reported in treating peripheral retinal tears, for postvitrectomy laser treatment of a giant retinal tear, and for treating proliferative diabetic retinopathy with panretinal photocoagulation. Treatment of macular lesions, such as choroidal neovascular membranes, should be avoided if possible, since the surgeon has less control over patient eye movement. A clear lens without yellow coating should be used to avoid absorption of the laser by the yellow tint.

COMMONLY USED LENSES FOR ANTERIOR SEGMENT LASER SURGERY

The Abraham iridectomy lens has been the lens of choice for creating a laser peripheral iridectomy. It employs a modified Goldmann-type fundus lens with a flat glass plate bonded to its anterior surface. A +66 D button is bonded into a decentered 8 mm hole that has been trephined into the periphery. This button creates a laser spot on the iris that is one-half the diameter of the spot that otherwise would be created without it. The fourfold increase in power density on the surface of the iris with a corresponding fourfold decrease in power density at the surface of the cornea reduces the chances for a corneal burn.[1]

The Wise iridotomy–sphincterotomy laser lens employs the same principle of a high-plus button, except with more dioptric power (+103 D). The manufacturer claims that the energy delivered to the iris is almost 8 times greater than with a plano lens and nearly 3 times greater than with an Abraham lens. Greater precision is required to focus and treat the iris with this high dioptric power.[7]

The Goldmann fundus lens, with either a single mirror inclined at 62 degrees or the three-mirror style with the gonioscopy mirror angled at 59 degrees, provides a large field of view but must be rotated 360 degrees to view the angle structures.[1] The single-mirror style has a small diameter, which makes for easy lens manipulation. The relatively bulky three-mirror lens can be found either with or without a flange for stability, and there are smaller sizes for pediatric use.

Suture cutting can be performed safely with the laser using a Hoskins nylon suture laser lens whose polymethyl methacrylate flange compresses the conjunctiva overlying the suture.[8] A 3.0 mm biconvex glass button centered in the flange allows a finely focused laser beam to sever the nylon suture. This laser technique can be useful in the postoperative management of cataract or trabeculectomy surgery.

COMMONLY USED LENSES FOR POSTERIOR SEGMENT LASER SURGERY

The Hruby lens is a high minus (originally −58.6 D), noncontact lens mounted on the slit lamp for stability. It provides a high-resolution, upright image of structures in the posterior pole, although the small field of view makes it difficult to be certain of the relationship of nearby structures. Visualization of more peripheral structures is limited by the entrance pupil, which is minified by the negative optics. This lens should be used only for observation purposes and not laser surgery.

The +90 D lens has gained favor recently as a diagnostic lens because it is a noncontact lens that avoids the inconvenience of contact lens solutions

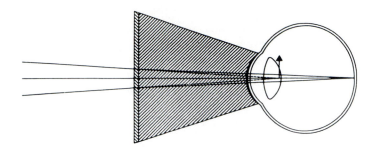

Figure 2–1. The Goldmann lens has a flat anterior surface and produces an erect, virtual ophthalmoscopic image located near the posterior surface of the crystalline lens. *(From Mainster MA, Crossman JL, Erickson PJ, Heacock GL: Retinal laser lenses: magnification, spot size, and field of view. Br J Ophthalmol 1990; 74:177-179, with permission.)*

and potential compromise in corneal clarity. After a minimum amount of time to become familiar with manipulation of the lens, the similarities to indirect ophthalmoscopy are apparent. The relatively wide field of view and good resolution are features that make the lens popular. However, it should not replace a fundus contact lens for determination of fluid in the macula. Subtle amounts of clinically significant fluid often associated with a choroidal neovascular membrane or central serous choroidopathy may be missed while using a +90 D lens.

Lenses that require saline or viscous solutions for corneal contact are preferred for posterior segment laser photocoagulation (Figs. 2–1 to 2–4, Table 2–1). The premier contact type of lens is the Goldmann fundus lens (−64 D), which is considered the standard for macular work. The lens produces an erect, virtual image located near the posterior surface of the crystalline lens, with excellent magnification.

The Yannuzzi lens is a modification of an earlier model developed by Krieger in 1966, designed to facilitate macular photocoagulation.[9] Besides having theoretically better optics than a simple Goldmann fundus lens, the concave corneal surface is steeper and of greater diameter. This allows posterior lens pressure to be transmitted to the sclera without distorting the cornea. Posterior pressure on the lens improves control of the eye when not using a retrobulbar block and is a useful maneuver to blanch choroidal vessels in case of a puncture of Bruch's membrane from too intense photocoagulation.

The Goldmann three-mirror lens is another standard lens for viewing and treating the posterior pole and periphery. By employing three progressively

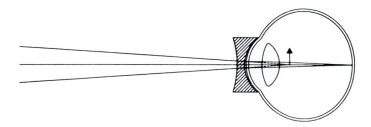

Figure 2–2. The Krieger lens has a concave anterior surface and produces an erect, virtual ophthalmoscopic image located in the anterior vitreous humor. *(From Mainster MA, Crossman JL, Erickson PJ, Heacock GL: Retinal laser lenses: magnification, spot size, and field of view. Br J Ophthalmol 1990; 74:177–179, with permission.)*

TABLE 2–1. OPHTHALMOSCOPIC LASER CONTACT LENSES

Parameter	Goldmann[a]	Krieger[b]	Panfundoscope[c]	Mainster[b]
Anterior surface	Flat	Concave, spherical	Convex, spherical	Convex, aspherical
Power[d]	−67	−92	+85	+61
Image type	Virtual, erect	Virtual, erect	Real, inverted	Real, inverted
Image location	Posterior capsule	Vitreous humor	Biconvex lens	Air

[a]Haag-Streit, Bern, Switzerland.
[b]Ocular Instruments, Bellevue, WA.
[c]Rodenstock, Munich, West Germany.
[d]Refractive power in diopters of the entire ophthalmoscopic lens system in air, as determined from direct measurement.
From Mainster MA, Crossman JL, Erickson PJ, Heacock GL: Retinal laser lenses: magnification, spot size, and field of view. Br J Ophthalmol *1990; 74:177-179, with permission.*

steeper internal reflecting surfaces (59 degrees for gonioscopy and the ora serrata if the view permits, 67 degrees for the ora to the equator, and 73 degrees for the equator to the posterior pole) and rotating the lens to scan circumferentially, the retina can be viewed almost in its entirety.[1] However, this requires the integration of multiple small fields of view. The chief disadvantage of the Goldmann lens is its small field of view, which prompted the development of other lenses.

The Rodenstock panfunduscopic lens (Fig. 2–3), introduced in 1969 by Schlegel, is an excellent lens for performing panretinal photocoagulation from the posterior pole to beyond the equator without the use of mirrors. It is useful for diagnosing complex vitreoretinal relationships when a panoramic view is desirable, which also translates into greater safety when performing panretinal ablation, since the key landmarks of the optic disc and temporal arcades are easy to find in this lens. The panfunduscopic lens produces an inverted, real image located in its spherical biconvex anterior lens element. Thus, the biomicroscope must be located further from the patient's eye than when using a Goldmann lens. Low biomicroscopic magnification produces adequate magnification, with a large field and acceptable depth of focus. The greater working field of the panfunduscopic lens (84% greater than a Goldmann), however, is at the expense of less lateral magnification (24% less than a Goldmann)[10] (Table 2–2). Increased biomicroscopic magnification cannot compensate for this loss, so for precision work, such as treating choroidal neovascular membranes, a Goldmann-type fundus lens is mandatory. The spot size on the retina is by one calculation 40% larger than the photocoagulator setting, whereas clinical opinion suggests that the size increase is twice that of a conventional contact lens.[11,12]

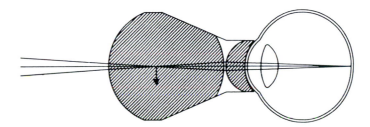

Figure 2–3. The panfundoscope lens has a biconvex, spherical anterior lens element and produces an inverted, real image inside the biconvex lens. *(From Mainster MA, Crossman JL, Erickson PJ, Heacock GL: Retinal laser lenses: magnification, spot size, and field of view.* Br J Ophthalmol *1990; 74:177-179, with permission.)*

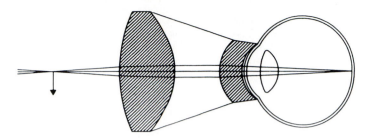

Figure 2–4. The Mainster lens has a biconvex, aspherical anterior lens element and produces an inverted, real image anterior to the biconvex lens. *(From Mainster MA, Crossman JL, Erickson PJ, Heacock GL: Retinal laser lenses: magnification, spot size, and field of view. Br J Ophthalmol 1990; 74:177-179, with permission.)*

The Mainster lens (Fig. 2–4), introduced in 1986, was designed to overcome the small field of the Goldmann three-mirror lens and the lesser magnification of the panfunduscopic lens. Like the panfunduscopic lens, it produces an inverted, real image, though located anterior to its biconvex and aspherical anterior lens element. This more anteriorly displaced image may require that the patient's head be moved posteriorly to accommodate a biomicroscope of limited travel. The Mainster lens has an intermediate working field (58% greater than a Goldmann but smaller than that of a panfunduscopic lens).[10] It has, however, excellent lateral and axial magnification, which makes the Mainster lens useful for detecting retinal thickening. It is thus a good choice for performing panretinal photocoagulation and focal diabetic macular work.

The Rodenstock panfunduscopic lens and Mainster lens have several features in common. Anterior segment irradiance becomes excessive with large spot sizes (1000 μm) but should be acceptable at a 500 μm spot size (Table 2–3). The field of view is increased in myopes and decreased in hyperopes and will lead to differences in how far peripherally laser photocoagulation can be applied[10] (Table 2–4). The experienced laser surgeon can achieve a more peripheral view by tilting the lens off-axis.

The Volk QuadrAspheric fundus lens is a newly introduced lens that attempts to improve on the aforementioned lens designs. The four aspheric surfaces of the two-element lens design also employs high-efficiency antireflection coatings. This purportedly improves lens performance by reducing astigmatism across the entire field of view and enhances visualization through a small pupil.[13] Oblong burns often occur when treating through the periphery of the Rodenstock panfunduscopic lens. Laser surgeons should be aware of the fact that an inverted and reversed image is created by the +60 D and +90 D lenses. This is similar to the image produced by the Rodenstock, Mainster, and Volk QuadrAspheric lenses.

TABLE 2–2. MAGNIFICATION AND FIELD OF VIEW FOR LASER OPHTHALMOSCOPIC CONTACT LENSES

Parameter	Goldmann	Krieger	Panfundoscope	Mainster
Lateral magnification	+0.93	+0.66	−0.71	−0.96
Relative magnification	1.00	0.71	0.76	1.03
Axial magnification	0.86	0.43	0.51	0.92
Instantaneous field of view[a]	±18°	±21°	±60°	±45°
Working field of view (with 15° tilt)[a]	±38°	±41°	±70°	±60°

[a]Half-field angle.
From Mainster MA, Crossman JL, Erickson PJ, Heacock GL: Retinal laser lenses: magnification, spot size, and field of view. Br J Ophthalmol 1990; 74:177-179, with permission.

TABLE 2–3. LASER BEAM DIAMETER AT CORNEA, LENS, AND RETINA VS PHOTOCOAGULATOR SPOT SIZE SETTING, FOR LASER BEAM FOCUSED ON RETINA[a]

Tissue (posterior surface)	Spot size setting (μm)	Tissue spot size (μm)			
		Goldmann	Krieger	Panfundoscope	Mainster
Cornea	100	1335	979	959	1285
	200	1321	1004	866	1164
	500	1432	1187	703	960
	1000	1793	1616	567	804
Lens	100	1048	791	760	1000
	200	1071	857	733	941
	500	1256	1138	742	887
	1000	1697	1700	859	934
Retina	100	108	153	141	105
	200	216	306	282	210
	500	541	764	704	524
	1000	1081	1529	1409	1048

[a]For example, with the laser beam focused on the retina and a 1000 μm photocoagulator spot size setting, beam diameter with panfundoscope lens will be 567 μm, 859 μm, and 1409 μm at the posterior surfaces of the cornea, lens, and retina respectively.
From Mainster MA, Crossman JL, Erickson PJ, Heacock GL: Retinal laser lenses: magnification, spot size, and field of view. Br J Ophthalmol 1990; 74:177-179, with permission.

TABLE 2–4. CHANGE IN MAGNIFICATION AND WORKING FIELD OF VIEW IN PATIENTS WITH AXIAL MYOPIA AND HYPEROPIA

Parameter	Goldmann	Krieger	Panfundoscope	Mainster
Magnification (myope, −3 D)	0	−1.5%	−4.2%	−5.2%
Magnification (hyperope, +3 D)	0	0	+5.6%	+4.2%
Field of view (myope, −3 D)	+5.3%	+4.9%	+8.6%	+6.7%
Field of view (hyperope, +3 D)	−5.3%	−2.4%	−5.7%	−6.7%

From Mainster MA, Crossman JL, Erickson PJ, Heacock GL: Retinal laser lenses: magnification, spot size, and field of view. Br J Ophthalmol 1990; 74:177-179, with permission.

SUMMARY

Selection of the proper lens for a particular task is a compromise between the individual's experience with his or her old lenses and the need to keep abreast of relevant, new technological developments in lens design and treatment strategy.

The author has no patent rights or other proprietary interests in the aforementioned lenses.

REFERENCES

1. Dieckert JP, Mainster MA, Ho PC: Contact lenses for laser applications. *Ophthalmology* 1984; (Instrument and Book suppl): 79–87.
2. Moffett DG Jr: A new lubricant (carboxymethylcellulose) for contact lens examination. *Arch Ophthalmol* 1991;109:173.
3. Gass JDM: Saline for contact lens ophthalmoscopy and photocoagulation. *Am J Ophthalmol* 1989;108:742.
4. Lundberg C: Biomicroscopic examination of the ocular fundus with a +60-diopter lens. *Am J Ophthalmol* 1985;99:490–491.
5. Whitacre MM: Noncontact retinal photocoagulation at the slit-lamp biomicroscope. *Am J Ophthalmol* 1987;104:290–293.
6. Bartov E, Treister G: Laser treatment of the retinal periphery with the +90-diopter lens. *Am J Ophthalmol* 1990;109:107.

7. Frankhauser F, Rol P, Kwaniewska S: Optical aids and their application. *Int Ophthalmol Clin* 1990;30:123–129.

8. Hoskins HD Jr, Migliazzo C: Management of failing filtering blebs with the argon laser. *Ophthalmic Surg* 1984;15:731–733.

9. Yannuzzi LA, Slakter JS: Macula photocoagulation lens (Letter to the Editor). *Am J Ophthalmol* 1986;101:619–620.

10. Mainster MA, Crossman JL, Erickson PJ, Heacock GL: Retinal laser lenses: magnification, spot size, and field of view. *Br J Ophthalmol* 1990;74:177–179.

11. Lobes Jr LA, Benson W, Grand G: Panfunduscope contact lens for argon laser therapy. *Ann Ophthalmol* 1981;13:713–714.

12. Blankenship GW: Panretinal laser photocoagulation with a wide-angle fundus contact lens. *Ann Ophthalmol* 1982;14:362–363.

13. Barker FM, Wing JT: Ultrawide field fundus biomicroscopy with the Volk quadraspheric lens. *J Am Optom Assoc* 1990;61:573–575.

CHAPTER 3

Clinicopathologic Correlation of Retinal Photocoagulation in the Human Eye

Ingolf Wallow

INTRODUCTION

The role of retinal photocoagulation has increased vastly over the last decade, particularly because of its successful application in the management of diabetic retinopathy. Photocoagulation, especially the diffuse or scatter modality, has become an effective retardant in proliferative diabetic retinopathy, as focal or grid photocoagulation has proven useful in nonproliferative retinopathy. The clinical end point for treatment always has been the ophthalmoscopic appearance of a fresh burn that has been correlated with the histopathologically defined amount of initial injury to the retina and choroid. Clinicopathologic correlations of the chronic stage of lesions have provided additional information.[1]

In the human eye, the clinical and histopathologic state of photocoagulation is well known for the acute stage (minutes to several days after exposure). However, comparable information for the chronic stage (approximately 3

15

weeks to months and years after exposure) is lacking because of the dearth of suitable tissue for examination. This pertains to both the currently used standard argon laser treatment and the older xenon arc modality.

Apple and associates[2] correlated physical parameters with histopathology when attempting to occlude retinal blood vessels with argon laser irradiation. Mild burns coagulated the outer part of the retina but spared the blood vessels. Moderate burns destroyed all of the retina but still did not result in vascular occlusion. Intense burns disrupted the retina, creating retinal detachments. These conclusions were based on examination of one eye. The burns were 1 day old, and the lesions were approximately 100 μm diameter spot size.

Weingeist[3] was concerned about the susceptibility of the nerve fiber layer in the papillomacular bundle. He found that photocoagulation of four eyes with 1-day-old lesions of 50 to 500 μm spot size was possible without destruction of the nerve fiber layer if the lesions were directed away from blood vessels and were mild. Mild lesions were defined as ophthalmoscopically just visible and involving morphologic damage of the outer half of the retina and of the inner nuclear layer.

Wallow and colleagues[4] were interested mainly in threshold lesions creating just visible burns that destroyed only the outer retina. Their results were consistent with Weingeist's conclusion that the nerve fiber layer can be spared. One eye with 1-day-old lesions of less than 50 μm spot size was used in this study.

Xenon arc photocoagulation burns have been investigated more extensively in human eyes. Curtin and Norton[5] produced light and heavy burns in three eyes and observed them at 2, 6, and 8 days. Light burns involved mainly the pigment epithelium. Heavy burns destroyed the entire retina, with inner limiting membrane involvement. The burns were unusually large, having a 6 degree diameter, as indicated on the photocoagulation machine. Blair and Gass[6] carried their observation time on one eye up to the 40 day chronic stage. Burns with a 3 degree diameter, initially white, did not demonstrate a loss of the structural integrity of the nerve fiber layer.

Lund[7] and Vogel[8] studied 43 and 54 eyes, respectively, at various stages during the acute and chronic periods after photocoagulation. The lesions were intended to destroy malignant melanomas of the choroid and were, therefore, heavier than lesions typically produced in scatter treatment of the retina. Immediately white burns obliterated the full thickness of the retina and caused atrophic scars on both the retina and the inner part of the choroid.

Studies on xenon arc burns have suffered from limitations similar to the argon studies quoted. Physical parameters of spot size and burn exposure times were not typical of most currently employed photocoagulation, and observation times usually were restricted to the acute stage. In addition, there was no consistent definition of lesions at both the clinical and histopathologic levels. Tso and co-workers[9] attempted to provide a more comprehensive classification by evaluating serial sections of 38 burns in eight human eyes. Clinical and histopathologic appearance were systematically correlated, classifying lesions into grades I, II, and III. Briefly, grade I lesions are not used as therapeutic burns. Grade II lesions involve approximately the outer half of the retina. They were not chosen for the typical scatter treatment in the Diabetic Retinopathy Study, nor are they typically employed in current scatter photocoagulation treatment. Grade III lesions are most commonly used yet cover a spectrum ranging from burns that involve the inner nuclear layer to those involving the internal limiting membrane and cortical vitreous. The concept of the study rested on the observation that with long clinical exposure times (100–500 msec or longer), conduction of heat laterally and vertically within the retina causes a pyramid of damage with its base at the retinal pigment epithelium (RPE) and its apex within the neurosensory retina. Retinal damage up to certain levels of the pyramid was then correlated with characteristic ophthalmoscopic appearances (Fig. 3–1). Tso and associates[9] and Wallow and colleagues[10] limited burn observation time to 3 days. Thus, the need remained to further define the spectrum of clinical lesions by describing the long-term results of such burns in humans.

Over the past 15 years, we have established and used a coordinated eye donor program in collaboration with the local eye bank. Retina clinic patients were informed about the opportunity to enroll in this program and to offer their eyes for corneal grafting or microscopic study after death. Many patients responded favorably, enabling us to collect a large number of eyes photocoagulated for various stages of diabetic retinopathy. Extensive preceding clinical information and photographic documentation often was available. This chapter presents a systematic summary of our observations that will fill some of the gaps of information described previously.

PATIENTS AND METHODS

Postmortem eyes were obtained and compared with clinical photographs. Ocular tissue was processed for light and electron microscopy. Individual and confluent argon laser and xenon arc photocoagulation lesions of varying

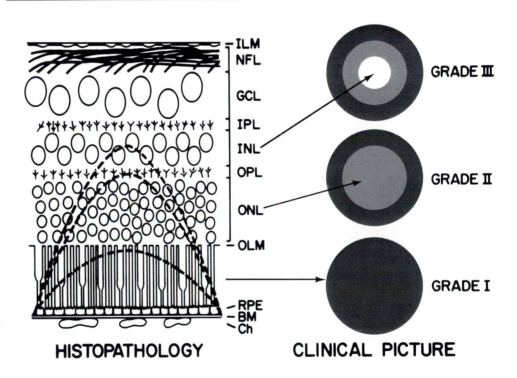

Figure 3–1. Schematic diagram illustrating the extent of retinal damage and the ophthalmoscopic appearance of three grades of retinal photocoagulation burns during their acute stage. The three dotted lines in the schematic histopathologic cross-section of the retina (**left**) demarcate the underlying extent of retinal necrosis of grade I, II, and III burns, respectively from bottom. The grade III burn shown involves just the inner nuclear layer and corresponds to a mild grade III lesion. Ch, choroid; BM, Bruch's membrane; RPE, retinal pigment epithelium; OLM, outer limiting membrane; ONL, outer nuclear layer, OPL, outer plexiform layer; INL, inner nuclear layer; IPL, inner plexiform layer; GCL, ganglion cell layer; NFL, nerve fiber layer; ILM, inner limiting membrane. Shaded areas in the schematic representation of the clinical picture (**right**) indicate zones of whitish retinal discoloration.

severity and age were dissected, evaluated, and measured according to a prescribed protocol.[11] Smaller tissue portions were embedded in an epoxy resin, and larger ones were embedded in glycol methacrylate or epoxy resin. All lesions were sectioned serially at 1.5 μm and stained with toluidine blue. Electron microscopic evaluation followed standard techniques of processing, sectioning, and staining.

Single photocoagulation burns are described according to their grade I, II, or III (Fig. 3–1) and acute and chronic stages are correlated by their ophthalmoscopic and histopathologic appearances. This is followed by an assessment of the clinical implications of each burn category. Since detailed photographic demonstrations of the ophthalmoscopic, light, and electron microscope appearances have been published elsewhere,[1–4,9–11,14–18] most illustrations for this chapter are schematic drawings.

Grade I Lesions

For the acute stage, correlations in humans were described from xenon arc burns of 3 degree spot size.[9,10] The burns were produced in patients with malignant tumors of the choroid before enucleation. For the chronic stage, extensive information has been obtained from experimental animals, mainly monkeys.

In the *acute stage*, grade I lesions ophthalmoscopically show an oval to round zone of barely visible grayish white retinal discoloration in the deeper part of the retina (Fig. 3–1). Histopathologically, damage is confined to the choriocapillaris, RPE, and photoreceptor elements (Fig. 3–1). There is a gradation of damage from the periphery to the center.

At the periphery, the cytoplasm of some endothelial cells of the choriocapillaris is swollen and discontinuous. Mononuclear cells containing lysosomes and cellular debris are seen outside the lumen of the choriocapillaris external and internal to Bruch's membrane, as they apparently are migrating into the subretinal space. Bruch's membrane is continuous. There is swelling of the RPE, with numerous cytoplasmic vacuoles and common gross disruption of the apical cytoplasm. Tubular and vesicular breakdown of the outer segments of rod cells and densification of the lamellae of cone outer segments are noted. The inner segments are swollen and occasionally contain discs of outer segments arranged in short stalks.

At the center of the lesions, discontinuities of the endothelium of the choriocapillaris are broad. Thrombotic material frequently fills the lumina. Bruch's membrane persists, and fibrin is noted within its connective tissue portion. The RPE shows densification and disintegration. Changes of the photoreceptor elements are more extensive than in the periphery.

The *chronic stage* of very small grade I lesions was studied in cynomolgus monkeys after argon laser exposure to minimal spot size. Ophthalmoscopically, there is a very subtle pigment mottling of the deep retina (Fig. 3–2). Histologically, the choriocapillaris is open, Bruch's membrane is intact, and the RPE has been repaired by a monolayer of hypopigmented cells. Outer segments are restored in the periphery of the lesion, and at the center, there is occasional dropout of inner segments and of photoreceptor cell nuclei. At times, pigment-laden or unpigmented macrophages are located in the subretinal space.[12] Cone cells seem more susceptible to photocoagulation damage than do rod cells.[13]

Clinical Significance. The clinical significance of grade I lesions is uncertain. They are not used intentionally in current ophthalmologic practice other than as test burns for safely approaching more intense lesions. Grade I lesions occlude the choriocapillaris only transiently during the acute stage, and dur-

GRADE I

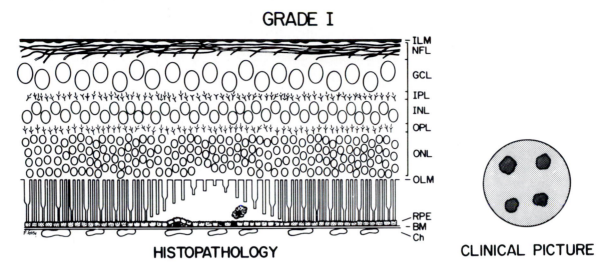

HISTOPATHOLOGY   CLINICAL PICTURE

Figure 3–2. Chronic stage of grade I photocoagulation burn.

ing later repair, the choriocapillaris becomes reestablished. The pigment epithelium is debrided but later replenished, probably by cell sliding and mild proliferation. Few photoreceptor cells are permanently missing. If debridement of the RPE alone were a therapeutic goal, grade I lesions would be ideal for that purpose, but they would be difficult to produce practically with any consistency.

Grade II Lesions

During the *acute stage,* lesions appear clinically as a grayish white ring around a denser whitish center (Fig. 3–1). Histopathologically, the grayish white ring corresponds to the damage seen in grade I lesions—that is, there is tissue destruction centering around the level of the RPE and photoreceptor elements. The denser, whitish center corresponds to tissue destruction exceeding the grade I level and extending into the outer nuclear and outer plexiform layers. Again, there is gradually increasing tissue involvement as the lesion is approached from its far periphery toward the paracentral region and into the center. Since the peripheral zone has been described under grade I lesions, the following comments refer only on the center.

The choriocapillaris is occluded by thrombi, and there is necrosis of endothelial cells, with massive outpouring of fibrin into Bruch's membrane and underneath the RPE. Bruch's membrane remains continuous. The pigment epithelial cells show pale, pyknotic nuclei or pale-staining nuclei that have lost their nuclear membrane. There is granulation of the cytoplasm and an irregular arrangement of the pigment granules. The photoreceptor outer and inner segments are necrotic, densely stained, and shrunken. The outer limiting membrane is poorly defined. Macrophages are frequent within the subretinal space. There are pyknosis and karyorrhexis of the nuclei of the outer layer. Rod and cone synapses are disrupted. The inner nuclear layer and the rest of the inner retina are spared from damage.

Grade II burns in their *chronic stage* appear ophthalmoscopically as a central brown ring containing some pigment mottling, surrounded by a grayish yellow hypopigmented periphery. Outside the lesion, a zone of mild, even hyperpigmentation is frequent. This zone is not shown in Figure 3–3.

GRADE II

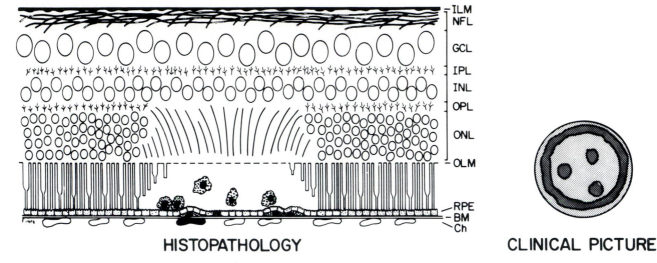

HISTOPATHOLOGY   CLINICAL PICTURE

Figure 3–3. Chronic stage of grade II photocoagulation burn.

Histopathologically in monkeys, there is the differentiated retinal repair already observed in grade I lesions. Testing with the tracers, horseradish peroxidase and fluorescein, shows that the pigment epithelial barrier of grade II lesions often is restored.[14] In addition, the outer limiting membrane is restored by hypertrophic Müller cells, producing zonulae adherentes arranged in a single plane. Most photoreceptor cells have disappeared, leaving a measurable defect in the outer nuclear layer.

In monkeys, single or confluent burns of 50 μm diameter had a restored RPE barrier 5 ½ weeks to 5 ½ months after argon laser photocoagulation (50 mW power, 0.2 sec exposure time). Half of the single 100 μm diameter burns and up to one third of confluent 100 μm burns (80 mW power, 0.2 sec exposure time) showed similar restoration. Underneath the RPE there was partial obliteration of the choriocapillaris. This has been confirmed by scanning electron microscopy of plastic injected vascular casts.[15] More subtle changes consist of reduction in number or absence of fenestrations in the endothelial cells of the choroidal capillaries.[16]

The first clinicopathologic correlation of focal argon laser treatment of human diabetic macular edema was evaluated for 50 μm to 100 μm spot size lesions at 0.1 sec exposure time.[17] Burns were observed clinically in their acute and chronic stages and histopathologically more than 3 years after exposure. Most burns fit into the category of grade II burns, but a few were more intense and represented mild grade III lesions. Some grade II burns in humans, in contrast to those in monkeys, showed incomplete repair of the outer limiting membrane, with hypertrophic Müller cells expanding into the subretinal and subpigment epithelial spaces. Müller glial cells then contributed fibrous membranes that extended far beyond the clinically visible edges of the burns.

Clinical Significance. Grade II burns will occlude permanently some of the choriocapillaris and debride the RPE transiently, yet frequently the RPE barrier is restored. Both occluded capillaries of the choroid and the restored RPE barrier may explain the clinical success of grade II lesions in central serous choroidopathy. Grade II lesions will also eliminate, over a short distance, the photoreceptor cell layer and create a new subretinal space lacking structural adhesion between the neurosensory retina and pigment epithelium. Such burns are not suitable for the treatment of retinal tears.[18] When applied for focal or grid photocoagulation of the macula, for example, in diabetic macular edema, such burns may affect diabetic lesions of the inner retina only indirectly. When placed too close to the center, they may endanger the fovea by giving rise to expanding subpigment epithelial fibrous membranes.

Grade III Lesions

Grade III lesions, which are used most commonly clinically, comprise a spectrum of burns arbitrarily divided into three categories: mild, moderate, and severe. They are defined according to the zonal pattern of retinal discoloration apparent shortly after exposure (Fig. 3–4). There is no significant clinical or histopathologic difference between similarly applied xenon arc and argon laser burns.

Mild Grade III Lesions

The *acute stage* ophthalmoscopic appearance differs from grade II burns by showing, within the more dense whitish zone, a distinct white center measuring less than one third of the entire burn diameter. The white center is associated with two surrounding rings, a whitish zone corresponding to grade II changes and a grayish peripheral zone corresponding to grade I changes (Fig. 3–1).

Histopathologically, the white center corresponds to necrosis of inner retinal layers, starting in the inner nuclear and inner plexiform layer. Choroidal and deep retinal changes are quantitatively more extensive than in grade II lesions. Bruch's membrane remains a continuous structure.

The *chronic stage* of all grade III lesions has been studied extensively in diabetic eyes 4 months to 6 years after scatter photocoagulation.[11,19] Ophthalmoscopically, mild grade III lesions contain a small core that shows continuous or mottled hyperpigmentation and is surrounded by a hypopigmented periphery (Fig. 3–5).

Histopathologically, the lesions obliterate part of the choriocapillaris and show scarring and hypopigmentation of the superficial choroid. At the periphery of the scars, healing of the RPE and of the neurosensory retina is identical to that of grade I and II lesions. Toward the center, RPE proliferation is pronounced, assuming the configuration of papillary trees.[20] The latter often join a glial retinal scar via zonula adherens junctions between RPE and glial cells (right side of histopathologic diagram in Fig. 3–5). Cells of the glial scar contact Bruch's membrane in areas where RPE proliferation is absent (left side of histopathologic diagram in Fig. 3–5). Pigment-laden macrophages are present among the proliferated RPE cells and within the retinal glial scar. The distribution of pigmented macrophages corresponds well with the pigmentation observed ophthalmoscopically. Defects in outer and inner nuclear layers measured 450 and 300 μm, respectively, at the center of argon laser burns produced by a 500 μm spot size at 500 mW to 800 mW power and 0.1 sec exposure time within lightly pigmented paracentral human retina.[11] Occasional ganglion cells and nerve fibers also are involved due to some variability of retinal thickness, retinal pigmentation, ocular media transparency, and exposure parameters. The superficial nerve fiber layer and the inner limiting membrane remain continuous.

Clinical Significance. Mild grade III lesions will eliminate larger areas of oxygen-demanding photoreceptor cells and nutrition-providing choroidal capillaries while preserving the inner aspect of the retinal architecture and the retinal thickness. Deep microaneurysms, typically located at the border

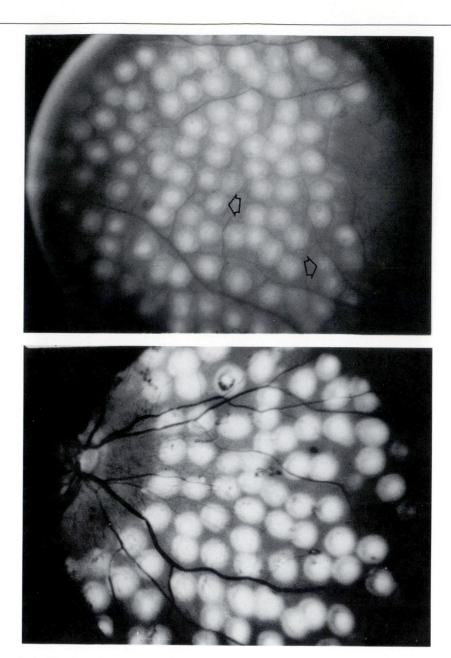

Figure 3–4. Fundus photographs of argon laser burns, 500 μm spot size, produced as scatter photocoagulation in two diabetic patients. **Top.** A few mild grade III burns (*arrows*), but most burns are moderate grade III lesions. Exposure time was 0.5 sec. and power was 320 mW. **Bottom.** Most burns in this field are severe grade III lesions. Exposure time was 0.5 sec, and power was 450 mW. The burns shown were produced 10 years ago. Currently, shorter exposure times of 0.1 sec or 0.2 sec are preferred, which allow less thermal conduction.

between the inner nuclear layer and outer plexiform layer, will be obliterated. Intraretinal microvascular abnormalities, usually located close to the inner retinal surface, likely will survive the direct photocoagulation effects. Some deeper fibers of the nerve fiber layer will be interrupted. Since the blood–retinal barrier at the RPE level will not be restored, substances leaving the scarred choroid can enter the retinal scar and the adjacent uninvolved retina. Morphologic retinopexies are frequent and focal in the peripheral retina but inconsistent in the thicker paracentral retina.

GRADE III (mild)

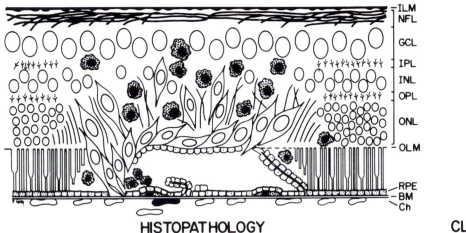

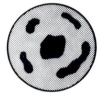

HISTOPATHOLOGY

CLINICAL PICTURE

Figure 3–5. Chronic stage of mild grade III photocoagulation burn.

Moderate Grade III Lesions

At the present time, these are the most frequently produced burns and may be ideal for scatter treatment. Ophthalmoscopically, they resemble mild grade III burns in their *acute stage*, except the white center measures up to approximately one half of the entire burn diameter, and the entire burn tends to be larger.

Histopathologically, the white center corresponds to an area of increasing damage to the inner retinal layers. The edge of the center shows necrosis of the inner nuclear and plexiform layers, and damage increases toward the middle of the burn to produce full-thickness retinal necrosis. The inner limiting membrane and the cuticular portion of Bruch's membrane persist as particularly resistant structures. In the choroid, there is widespread necrosis of vascular endothelial cells and of melanocytes, with extensive interstitial edema.

In the *chronic stage*, months to years after exposure, moderate grade III lesions typically appear as densely hyperpigmented central cores surrounded by a hypopigmented halo. The central hyperpigmented core is larger than in mild grade III burns. Although some lesions maintain this appearance indefinitely, others show a gradual decrease and irregularity of their central pigmentation with time (Fig. 3–6).

The histopathologic picture corresponds well with these ophthalmoscopic findings. In the choroid, obliteration of capillaries and formation of hypopigmented fibrous scars are more extensive. At times, open capillary lumens filled with plasma and red blood cells are seen next to the center of the burn, where damage must have been most severe. Presumably, some regeneration of small choroidal blood vessels takes place immediately adjacent to Bruch's membrane or within the superficial choroid. Bruch's membrane remains continuous. In the retina, papillary RPE proliferations are conspicuous, reach into the inner retina, and form a retinal scar together with glial cells. Proliferated RPE cells provide the bulk of the external part of the retinal scar, and extensive glial proliferation forms the internal part. The extent of RPE proliferation may vary, leaving gaps through which retinal glial cells prolapse toward Bruch's membrane. Light microscopic observations of 1.5 μm thick sections of the inner limiting membrane suggest that it usually remains a continuous structure. A detailed electron microscopic analysis is lacking.

GRADE III (moderate)

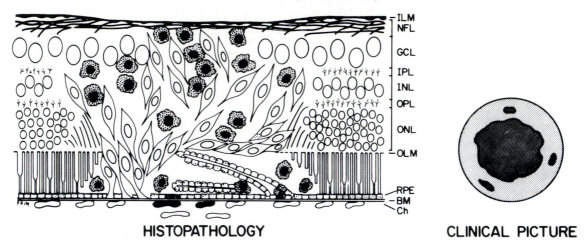

HISTOPATHOLOGY   CLINICAL PICTURE

Figure 3–6. Chronic stage of moderate grade III photocoagulation burn.

Pigment-laden macrophages are clustered throughout the scar but are more prominent in its inner aspect, that is, enmeshed among the glial cells. Often, they lie adjacent to the vitreous and are clearly visible and, thus, presumably account for the jet-black pigmentation of some scar centers. Gradual depigmentation in some lesions over the course of years may be explained by progressive atrophy of the scar and by retained ability of macrophages to leave the tissue they previously invaded. Retinal repair toward the periphery of the scars follows the pattern described for grade II and grade I lesions. Permanent retinal defects of 600 μm in diameter at the level of the outer nuclear layer and of 450 μm at the level of the inner nuclear layer were measured in argon laser burns of 500 μm spot size, approximately 500 mW power, 0.5 sec exposure time, applied to lightly pigmented diabetic retina.[11]

Clinical Significance. Moderate grade III lesions differ from mild grade III burns by consistently producing a central area of full-thickness retinal necrosis and by leading to a scar that thins the retina by approximately one third. It is unknown to what degree the vertical thinning of the retina is accompanied by lateral shrinkage. Retinopexies are broader than in mild grade III burns. New vessels on the retinal surface will not be affected so as to produce immediate thrombosis. Clinical experience, however, shows that new vessels frequently atrophy later, presumably via indirect effects that are not fully understood. Where active new vessels persist within areas treated by moderate grade III burns, direct retreatment can be rewarding. It has been feared that the hyperpigmentation of retinal scars will cause unpredictably high coagulation damage to the choroid, paving the way for chorioretinal feeder vessels and chorioretinovitreal neovascularization. Observations have shown that the scar tissue of moderate grade III lesions in front of Bruch's membrane remains quite thick. By using large spot sizes and long exposure times, several eyes have been rephotocoagulated successfully for persistent active new vessels, and vascular regression and atrophy have been achieved with only little and locally confined retinal traction and no chorioretinal neovascularization.

Ophthalmoscopically, in the *acute stage,* severe grade III burns show a white center extending over two thirds or more of the burn diameter. In addition, severe grade III burns are larger than other grade III lesions.

Histopathologically, they show full-thickness retinal necrosis over more than half of the burn diameter, with damage gradually decreasing toward the periphery according to the patterns described for less severe burns. The inner limiting membrane tends to retain continuity in the acute stage, but its final status needs further investigation. Macrophages are seen not only within the necrotic retina but also within the cortical vitreous along the inner limiting membrane. The extensive retinal damage and the presence of macrophages within the vitreous suggest that the cortical vitreous has received photocoagulation damage even though this may be difficult to assess morphologically. Posterior vitreous detachment may be facilitated. Bruch's membrane remains continuous in most burns, but rare disruption may occur, allowing hemorrhage in the acute stage and retinal invasion by chorioretinal feeder vessels later.[21] Endothelial necrosis of choroidal blood vessels and of choroidal melanocytes with dispersion of their pigment is widespread.

In the *chronic stage,* severe grade III lesions have a center consisting of a large depigmented core surrounded by a hyperpigmented ring. Peripheral changes resemble those of lighter burns (Fig. 3–7).

Histopathologically, in the center, the retinal repair by glial cells is minimal or absent and lacks pigment-laden macrophages. Only depigmented, proliferated RPE bridges the retinal gap over the central 300 μm. The retinal thickness is reduced by two thirds. The pigmented ring delineating the depigmented central core corresponds to a zone where the repair pattern of moderate grade III lesions begins. Glial cells contribute to the restoration and contain in their meshwork clumps of pigmented scavenger cells. In some severe grade III lesions, the inner limiting membrane cannot be traced by light microscopy. It is surprising to see that proliferated RPE remains confined to the level of the retina and is only rarely seen to invade the vitreous.[22] In diabetic patients treated for proliferative retinopathy, avascular glial preretinal membranes were present in front of two thirds of severe xenon arc burns but in front of only approximately one tenth of severe argon laser burns.[11] Bruch's membrane, with few exceptions, remains continuous. The scarred choroid

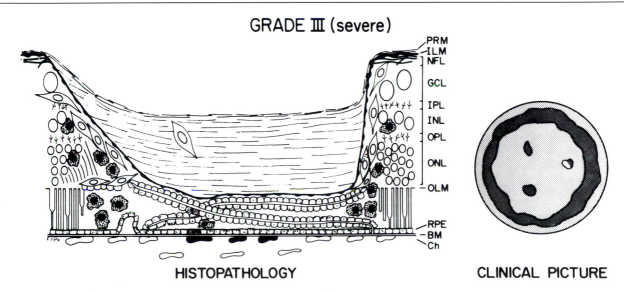

GRADE III (severe)

HISTOPATHOLOGY   CLINICAL PICTURE

Figure 3–7. Chronic stage of severe grade III photocoagulation burn. Note: PRM = fibrous preretinal membrane.

often becomes so avascular and depigmented that on clinical examination, it resembles sclera. Permanent retinal defects of approximately 900 μm in diameter at the level of the outer nuclear layer and 800 μm at the level of the inner nuclear layer were measured in argon laser burns of 500 μm spot size, up to 800 mW power, and 0.5 sec exposure time applied to lightly pigmented diabetic retina. Severe grade III xenon arc photocoagulation burns produced by a cone size of 4.5 degrees showed an almost identical extent of damage.[11]

Clinical Significance. Severe grade III lesions are, for the most part, undesirable and usually unnecessary. They tend to involve the cortical vitreous and were found to be associated with avascular preretinal membranes. In one case such a membrane produced wrinkling of the retinal surface, and later, the inner limiting membrane was found ruptured and recoiled.[19] On rare occasions, severe grade III lesions also will weaken the retinochoroidal interface, promoting the growth of chorioretinal or chorioretinovitreal neovascularization.[21] Advocacy of photocoagulation treatment for small choroidal tumors has been revived recently. Severe grade III lesions produced for the treatment of such tumors may cause misleading scars. The center of such burns in the chronic stage becomes depigmented and may resemble bare sclera. However, this is not a reliable sign that an underlying tumor has been destroyed. Instead, proliferated RPE and scarred choroid may prevent a deeper ophthalmoscopic view. Newer lasers emitting in the near infrared, such as the diode laser (810 nm), penetrate more deeply into the choroid and cause more profound choroidal scars.[23] Particularly if combined with photothermal or photochemical agents or both, these new lasers seem to offer a better chance of effectively treating small choroidal tumors. Among the useful effects of severe grade III lesions are extensive retinopexy and direct destruction of preretinal new vessels.[24] In cases where new vessels actively proliferate despite extensive use of standard scatter treatment, one has to balance risks and benefits of focal treatment using moderate grade III lesions with later focal retreatment vs immediate focal treatment using severe grade III burns.

SUMMARY

The experience-proven gradation of retinal photocoagulation burns by their ophthalmoscopic appearance shortly after exposure is confirmed and organized into a new classification based on clinicopathologic correlations. Pigmentary changes in old burns often are also characteristic and permit classification of the severity of the initial burns and of the configuration of the resulting scars. The proposed grading system is independent of such biologic variables as retinal thickness, pigmentation, and media transparency.

REFERENCES

1. Apple D: Histopathology of xenon arc and argon laser photocoagulation. In: L'Esperance FA, ed. *Current Diagnosis and Management of Chorioretinal Diseases.* St. Louis: CV Mosby; 1977:25–93.
2. Apple DJ, Goldberg MF, Wyhinny GJ: Histopathology and ultrastructure of the argon laser lesion in human retinal and choroidal vasculatures. *Am J Ophthalmol* 1973;75:595–609.
3. Weingeist TA: Argon laser photocoagulation of the human retina: I. Histopathologic correlation of chorioretinal lesions in the region of the maculopapillar bundle. *Invest Ophthalmol* 1974;13:1024–1032.
4. Wallow IHL, Lund OE, Gabel VP: A comparison of retinal argon laser lesions in

man and in cynomolgus monkey. *Graefes Arch Clin Exp Ophthalmol* 1974;189: 159–164.

5. Curtin VT, Norton EWD: Early pathological changes of photocoagulation in the human retina. *Arch Ophthalmol* 1963;69:744–751.
6. Blair CJ, Gass JDM: Photocoagulation of the macula and papillomacular bundle in the human. *Arch Ophthalmol* 1972;88:167–171.
7. Lund OE: Changes in choroidal tumors after light coagulation (and diathermy coagulation). *Arch Ophthalmol* 1966;75:458–466.
8. Vogel M: Histopathologic observations of photocoagulated malignant melanomas of the choroid. *Am J Ophthalmol* 1972;74:466–474.
9. Tso MOM, Wallow IHL, Elgin S: Experimental photocoagulation of the human retina: I. Correlation of physical, clinical and pathologic data. *Arch Ophthalmol* 1977;95:1035–1040.
10. Wallow IHL, Tso MOM, Elgin S: Experimental photocoagulation of the human retina: II. Electron microscopic study. *Arch Ophthalmol* 1977;95:1041–1050.
11. Wallow IHL, Davis MD: Clinicopathologic correlation of xenon arc and argon laser photocoagulation procedure in human diabetic eyes. *Arch Ophthalmol* 1979;97: 2308–2315.
12. Wallow IHL, Birngruber R, Gabel VP, Hillenkamp F, Lund OE: Netzhautreaktionen nach Intensivlichtbestrahlung: I. Schwellenläsionen. *Adv Ophthalmol* 1975; 31:159–232.
13. Tso MOM, Wallow IHL, Powell JO: Differential susceptibility of rod and cone cells to argon laser. *Arch Ophthalmol* 1973;89:228–234.
14. Wallow IHL: Repair of the pigment epithelial barrier following photocoagulation. *Arch Ophthalmol* 1984;102:126–135.
15. Perry DD, Risco M: Choroidal microvascular repair after argon laser photocoagulation. *Am J Ophthalmol* 1982;93:787–793.
16. Tso MOM, Wallow IHL, Powell JO, Zimmerman LE: Recovery of the rod and cone cells after photic injury. *Trans Am Acad Ophthalmol Otolaryngol* 1972;76:1247–1262.
17. Wallow IHL, Bindley CD: Focal photocoagulation of diabetic macular edema: a clinicopathologic case report. *Retina* 1988;8:261–269.
18. Wallow IHL, Tso MOM: Failure of formation of chorioretinal adhesions following xenon-arc photocoagulation: limitations and prospects for retinal surgery. *Mod Probl Ophthalmol* 1974;12:189–201.
19. Wallow IHL: Long-term changes in photocoagulation burns. *Dev Ophthalmol* 1981; 2:318–327.
20. Wallow IHL, Tso MOM: Proliferation of the retinal pigment epithelium over malignant choroidal tumors. *Am J Ophthalmol* 1972;73:914–926.
21. Wallow IHL, Johns K, Barry P, Chandra S, Bindley C: Chorioretinal and choriovitreal neovascularization after photocoagulation for proliferative diabetic retinopathy: a clinicopathologic correlation. *Ophthalmology* 1985;92:523–532.
22. Wallow IHL, Miller SA: Preretinal membrane by retinal pigment epithelium. *Arch Ophthalmol* 1978;96:1643–1646.
23. Wallow IHL, Sponsel WE, Stevens TS: Clinicopathologic correlation of diode laser burns in monkey. *Arch Ophthalmol* 1991;109:648–653.
24. Wallow IHL, Skuta GL: Histopathology of focally photocoagulated preretinal new vessels. *Arch Ophthalmol* 1984;102:1340–1344.

CHAPTER 4

Clinical Applications of Diabetic Retinopathy Studies

George H. Bresnick and Matthew D. Davis

INTRODUCTION

The Diabetic Retinopathy Study (DRS) was a randomized, controlled clinical trial sponsored by the National Eye Institute to evaluate photocoagulation treatment for proliferative diabetic retinopathy (PDR). Sixteen clinic centers participated, enrolling 1758 patients between June 1972 and September 1975. Follow-up was completed in June 1979.

The ultimate value of such a study depends primarily on the extent to which its results can be translated into everyday clinical practice, either supporting or altering existing guidelines for the care and prevention of a disease. With respect to the DRS, three general aspects of the results have had a significant impact on our understanding of and management approach to PDR:

(1) natural history of untreated eyes, and in particular the identification of certain high-risk characteristics that forebode a poor prognosis for the retention of vision, (2) beneficial effects of treatment, and (3) undesirable side effects of treatment. Armed with a knowledge of the prognostic significance of certain features of the retinopathy and with information regarding the potential benefits and risks of treatment, one can, in an informed and intelligent fashion, weigh the relative consequences of recommending prompt photocoagulation or of deferring treatment of a given eye. This provides the clinician with a secure foundation from which to make therapeutic decisions and provides the patient a rational base from which to give a truly informed consent.

One should be aware, at the outset, of certain caveats in applying DRS results to clinical practice. (1) The results apply to a particular sample of the diabetic population, which contained relatively few eyes with very severe PDR. (2) A standard treatment technique was used, and one cannot assume that other techniques would produce comparable results (although minor departures from the standard technique probably would do so). (3) Certain questions of importance in the treatment of PDR were not addressed in the DRS. First, the effect of photocoagulation on macular edema was not determined. Second, the DRS began by studying the relative value of immediate photocoagulation vs no photocoagulation treatment. The study protocol did not compare immediate treatment with judicious deferral of treatment. Therefore, although definite statements can be made regarding the value of "treatment now" vs "no treatment ever," the relative efficacy of restricting treatment of eyes with PDR to those with known high-risk characteristics and deferring treatment in eyes without these characteristics was not studied. After it became clear in 1976 that the beneficial effect of treatment in reducing the risk of severe visual loss outweighed the risk of harmful treatment effects for eyes with high-risk characteristics, the protocol was modified. Treatment of those eyes assigned initially to the control group in which high-risk characteristics had developed was recommended if treatment was still feasible.

NATURAL COURSE AND PATHOPHYSIOLOGY OF PROLIFERATIVE DIABETIC RETINOPATHY

Proliferative diabetic retinopathy always occurs against a background of the following nonproliferative intraretinal changes: (1) those due to increased retinal vascular permeability and (2) those due to retinal vascular occlusion. It is the retinal ischemia resulting from the latter that is thought to be the intraretinal stimulus for the preretinal proliferation of neovascular and fibrous tissue. An eye with nonproliferative retinopathy, in which severe signs of retinal ischemia develop, is considered to have entered a preproliferative phase because the eye is at high risk to develop fibrovascular proliferation.

The signs of retinal ischemia that are the most important harbingers of PDR are those due to retinal arteriolar obstruction. These include (1) cotton-wool spots (inner retinal layer ischemic infarcts), (2) beaded veins (dilated venous segments due to ischemia in the adjacent retina), (3) large, dark blot hemorrhages (hemorrhagic retinal infarcts), and (4) white, threadlike (occluded) arterioles. The new vessels tend to develop in spatial proximity to these sites of focal retinal ischemia.[1] One should realize, however, that retinal hemorrhages, cotton-wool spots, and dilated capillaries may fade remarkably before the new vessels develop. Thus, the retinal abnormalities may seem to be improving when, in fact, the eye is about to enter the more serious proliferative phase of the disease.

Two stages of PDR are recognized, a *proliferative stage,* in which new vessels and fibrous and glial tissue proliferate, and a *contraction stage,* in which the proliferative tissue, the vitreous, or both shrink to produce tractional complications.

Fibrovascular proliferation begins with the sprouting of neovascular tufts from the retinal vessels. The new vessels break through the internal limiting membrane of the retina and arborize at the interface between retina and vitreous. The vascular tufts during growth and extension most likely interdigitate with the collagen fibrils in the cortical vitreous, thereby producing an *adhesion* between the new vessels and the cortical vitreous. This adhesion becomes extremely important in the contraction stage of PDR. At the inception of proliferation, the neovascular frond is relatively naked, or free of fibrous tissue, but later the frond becomes more fibrotic. Ultimately, the frond evolves into a predominantly fibrous tissue network, and the new vessels become sclerotic.

During this initial proliferative stage, the fibrovascular tissue lies flat on the inner retina surface. Subsequent shrinkage of the fibrous tissue or the associated cortical vitreous or both during the contraction stage causes elevation of the fibrovascular tissue and may produce vitreous hemorrhage from the thin-walled new vessels. If the shrinkage is sufficiently severe, tractional detachment of the retina or distortion or lateral displacement of the retina also may develop.

Serious loss of vision in eyes with PDR can result from one or more of the following processes: (1) vitreous hemorrhages from preretinal new vessels, (2) tractional complications, including macular detachment, macular displacement (heterotopia), and macular distortion due to retinal wrinkling, and (3) obscuration of the macula by fibrous or glial tissue in the form of either epiretinal membranes or opacification of the detached posterior hyaloid face. Vision in eyes with PDR also may be reduced by intraretinal changes, most commonly macular edema and hard exudate deposition and macular ischemia. In determining the causes of visual loss in an eye with PDR, one should consider the different elements outlined previously and attempt to evaluate the relative contribution of each.

The natural course of PDR is extremely variable from one patient to another and even between the two eyes of a given patient. In many eyes, the disease progresses slowly, with mild new vessel and fibrous tissue growth. Most of these cases eventually develop visual symptoms for the reasons discussed previously, but a minority (probably less than 10%) undergo a spontaneous regression and remain free of symptoms. Other eyes, in contrast, develop rapid and severe proliferation of fibrovascular tissue, with subsequent vitreous hemorrhage and severe tractional complications. Identification at an early stage of those eyes that are destined to develop severe progressive changes would be of great value, but at the present time, this is not possible. One can, however, describe certain characteristic subgroups of retinopathy that do suggest a poor visual prognosis.

Florid Diabetic Retinopathy

In this subgroup, severe intraretinal changes precede and accompany the preretinal proliferative changes. Numerous dilated intraretinal capillaries [so-called intraretinal microvascular abnormalities (IRMA)], cotton-wool spots, beaded veins, and a wet retina (diffuse retinal edema) are present, indicative of active retinal ischemia (Fig. 4–1). The patient is usually a juvenile-onset diabetic in the 20 to 40-year age range. The onset of these intraretinal changes is often acute, both eyes are affected simultaneously, and progressive neovascularization develops rapidly. The course in such cases has been described as

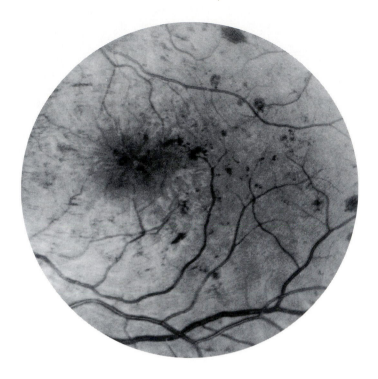

Figure 4–1. Florid diabetic retinopathy in a 25-year-old woman with insulin-dependent diabetes for 14 years. **A.** Left eye shows multiple dark blot retinal hemorrhages, dilated capillaries, and cystoid macular edema. Visual acuity 20/30. *(From Bresnick GH. Background diabetic retinopathy. In: Ryan SJ, Schachat AP, Murphy RB, Patz A, eds.* Retina. *St. Louis: CV Mosby Co.; 1989, with permission)*

"rapid, bloody, and blinding." Photocoagulation treatment frequently is ineffective but should be attempted. Since systemic hypertension and renal decompensation may accompany and perhaps contribute to this syndrome, the patient's systemic status should be evaluated, and abnormalities should be treated medically. In the past, some groups[2,3] have recommended pituitary ablation in such patients and claim a more favorable visual outcome than with photocoagulation. The morbidity of the procedure is too great, however, to warrant such a radical approach. Vitrectomy, performed before extensive contraction, when the response to photocoagulation is poor, or when photocoagulation is precluded by vitreous hemorrhage is an alternative approach that has been shown to be of benefit in eyes with very severe new vessels (see Diabetic Retinopathy Vitrectomy Study, to follow).

Severe Arteriolar Ischemia

Severe retinal arteriolar ischemia, with nonperfusion of extensive areas of retina and constriction of the visual field,[4] may develop in some eyes. If the macular blood supply is affected, as is often the case, severe loss of visual acuity (20/200 or worse) develops as well (Fig. 4–2). The fundus changes include retinal arteriolar narrowing and sclerosis, dark blot hemorrhages, and ultimately a dry (nonedematous) retina and optic disc pallor. Fibrovascular proliferation usually is present but is less severe than and is overshadowed by the retinal arteriolar obstructive changes. Such eyes frequently develop severe rubeosis iridis and neovascular glaucoma. There is suggestive evidence that

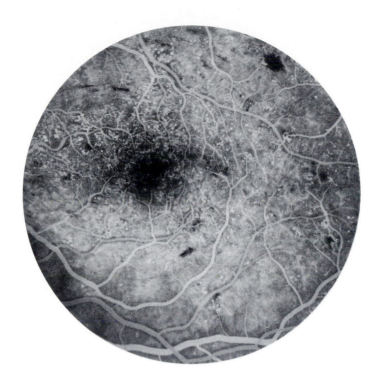

Figure 4–1 B. Fluorescein angiogram demonstrates diffusely dilated capillaries and extensive diffuse leakage from the capillary bed in the posterior pole. *(From Bresnick GH. Background diabetic retinopathy. In Ryan SJ, Schachat AP, Murphy RB, Patz A, eds. Retina. (St. Louis: CV Mosby Co.; 1989, with permission)*

extensive scatter photocoagulation may cause a severe posttreatment reduction in visual acuity[4] (Fig. 4–2C). Nonetheless, photocoagulation seems warranted because of the very poor prognosis without treatment.

Severe Fibrous Proliferation

In some eyes, the proliferation of fibrous tissue is unusually severe and rapid. The fibrous component of the fibrovascular fronds predominates, opacification and thickening of the detached posterior hyaloid across the posterior pole progress rapidly, and extensive epiretinal membrane formation may develop. Severe tractional complications are frequent in such eyes, and some observers have expressed concern that panretinal photocoagulation may exacerbate the fibrous tissue proliferation and contraction.

DIABETIC RETINOPATHY STUDY

Protocol

The efficacy of photocoagulation treatment in preventing severe visual loss in eyes with PDR was convincingly demonstrated in the Diabetic Retinopathy Study (DRS).[5–7] The DRS was a randomized, controlled collaborative clinical trial in which patients with proliferative retinopathy in at least one eye or severe nonproliferative retinopathy in both eyes had one eye randomly assigned to either xenon or argon photocoagulation and the opposite eye fol-

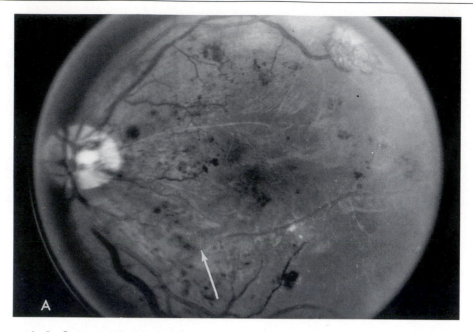

Figure 4–2. Severe retinal ischemia in a 30-year-old man with insulin-dependent diabetes for 27 years. **A.** Note white, threadlike vessels and optic disc pallor. Multiple large dark hemorrhages are present in the left side of the field, and absence of vascular pattern is noted on the right side. Note irregular caliber of macular branch of inferotemporal arteriole *(arrow)*. New vessels are present on the optic disc and along the superior temporal vein. *(From Bresnick et al: Retinal ischemia in diabetic retinopathy. Arch Ophthalmol 1975;93:1300–1310, with permission.)*

lowed without treatment. Other major eligibility criteria included visual acuity 20/100 or better in each eye, no previous photocoagulation in either eye, and both eyes suitable for photocoagulation. It should be noted that relatively few eyes with very severe proliferative retinopathy actually were entered in the study (Table 4–1). Although 80% of all eyes had new vessels on entry, only 10% of these had severe new vessels on or within 1 disc diameter of the disc (NVD), and only 5% had severe new vessels greater than 1 disc diameter from the disc (NVE, new vessels elsewhere). In addition, less than 5% of eyes had severe fibrous proliferation. Vitreous hemorrhage or preretinal hemorrhage was present in 25% of eyes. In applying the results of the DRS to clinical practice, one must keep in mind, therefore, that the majority of eyes studied were not in the very severe proliferative category.

The photocoagulation technique used in the DRS differed in some respects from the argon laser and xenon arc modalities (Table 4–2). In general, the strength of the argon laser treatment can be considered of moderate intensity, whereas the xenon treatment was more intense, with stronger, larger

TABLE 4–1. STAGES OF RETINOPATHY ACTUALLY ENROLLED IN THE DRS

DRS	% of Eyes with specified lesions
New vessels	80%
New vessels on or within 1 DD[a] of disc (NVD) severe	10%
New vessels > 1 DD from disc (elsewhere, NVE) severe	5%
Fibrous proliferations severe	<5%
Vitreous and/or preretinal hemorrhage (VH/PRH) present	25%

[a]DD, disc diameter.

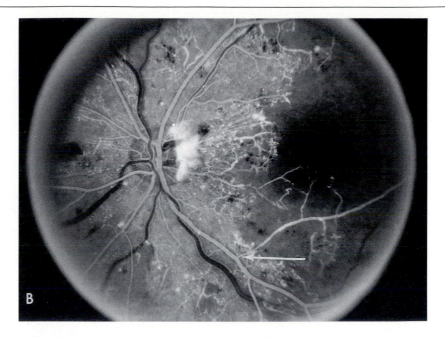

Figure 4–2B. Fluorescein angiogram showing extensive capillary nonperfusion in the temporal field and far nasal field. Dilated tortuous retinal vessels are seen in the papillomacular region. The blood supply to the macula is severely compromised. Visual acuity 20/50. Note narrowed fluorescein column at origin of inferotemporal arteriole (*arrow*). *(From Bresnick et al: Retinal ischemia in diabetic retinopathy. Arch Ophthalmol 1975;93:1300–1310, with permission.)*

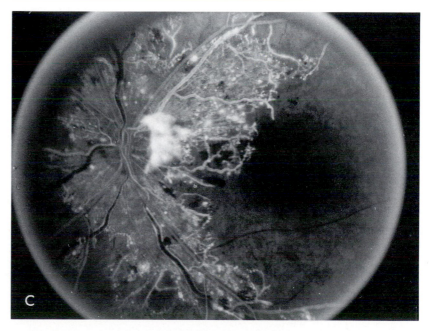

Figure 4–2C. Closure of inferotemporal arteriolar branch to the macula 19 days after panretinal photocoagulation treatment delivered in a single session. Visual acuity decreased from 20/50 to 20/200. *(From Bresnick et al: Retinal ischemia in diabetic retinopathy. Arch Ophthalmol 1975;93:1300–1310, with permission.)*

burns. In most eyes, all or most scatter (panretinal) burns were applied in a single sitting, in the numbers specified in Table 4–2. Direct treatment was applied to NVE on the surface of the retina in both argon and xenon techniques and to elevated NVE and to NVD in the argon technique only. The protocol specified follow-up treatment, direct or additional scatter or both, when new vessels failed to regress or when they recurred.

Benefits of Treatment

The major end point considered in the DRS was "severe visual loss," defined as visual acuity less than 5/200 at two consecutively completed follow-up visits (scheduled at 4-month intervals). A comparison of treated and untreated eyes revealed an overall reduction in the rate of severe visual loss of approximately 50% by photocoagulation. This was true whether observations were limited to those made under the original protocol or included those made after the protocol was changed in 1976 to encourage photocoagulation of some control group eyes (Fig. 4–3). When the results of xenon treatment were compared with those of argon treatment, the difference in rates of severe visual loss between treated and control eyes was slightly greater in the xenon treatment group (Fig. 4–4), but the greater frequency and severity of harmful treatment effects in this group outweighed this possible advantage.

As noted previously, the overall reduction of incidence of severe visual loss was about 50% when all eyes were considered. Since some undesirable side effects of treatment also were demonstrated, it was important to subdivide the eyes according to baseline retinopathy characteristics into those at high risk and those at lesser risk to develop severe visual loss without treatment. In those eyes at high risk, the undesirable side effects of treatment would be more acceptable because of the serious consequences of withholding treatment. In those eyes at lesser risk, side effects would be less acceptable, and deferral of treatment might be a reasonable alternative. Classification of eyes according to the location and severity of new vessels and presence or absence of vitreous or preretinal hemorrhage (VH/PRH) in baseline fundus photographs identified the following high-risk characteristics for severe visual loss without treatment.

NVD ≥ ⅓ disc area with or without VH/PRH
NVD < ⅓ disc area, with VH/PRH
NVE ≥ ½ disc area, with VH/PRH

The cumulative event rate of severe visual loss in these categories over a 2-year follow-up period is shown in Table 4–3. The event rate in some of the lower-risk categories is shown in Table 4–4.

A graph of the cumulative rates of severe visual loss (SVL) for eyes with and without high-risk characteristics, contrasting treated and untreated eyes, is shown in Figure 4–5. In all groups, the rate of severe visual loss in treated

TABLE 4–2. DRS PHOTOCOAGULATION TECHNIQUES

Scatter	Argon Moderate	Xenon Strong
Number of burns	800–1600 (500 μm) or 500–1000 (1000 μm)	400–800 (3°) or 200–400 (4.5°)
Focal		
surface NVE	+	+
Elevated NVE	+	−
NVD	+	−
Macular edema	+	+
Follow-up therapy	+	+

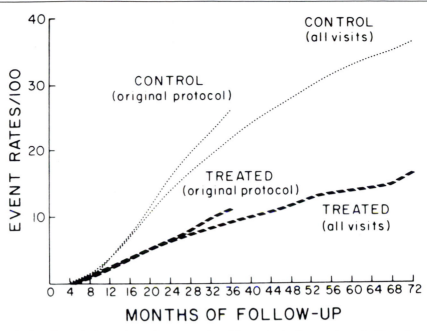

Figure 4–3. Cumulative rates of severe visual loss, including and excluding observations made after the 1976 protocol change, argon and xenon groups combined. *(Published courtesy of* Ophthalmology *1981;88:587.)*

eyes was less than 50% that in control eyes. However, because of the better visual prognosis in eyes without high-risk characteristics, it took a longer follow-up period before the 50% treatment effect became apparent. For example, in eyes with high-risk characteristics, the 50% reduction in SVL was apparent after only 1 year, in eyes with PDR without high-risk characteristics, it was apparent after 2 years, and in eyes with nonproliferative diabetic retinopathy (NPDR), it was not apparent until 3 years.

Risk of Treatment

The detrimental side effects of treatment were greater with xenon arc photocoagulation than with argon laser photocoagulation (Table 4–5). The side

TABLE 4–3. DRS: SEVERE VISUAL LOSS IN EYES WITH HRC AT INITIAL VISIT: TREATED VS UNTREATED EYES

Stage at Initial Visit	% of Eyes at 2 Year Visit with Visual Acuity $\leq$ 5/200		
	Control (n)	Treated (n)	Z^a
NVD $\geq$ 1/3 DA with VH/PRH[b]	36.9 (76)	20.1 (107)	3.2
NVD $\geq$ 1/3 DA without VH/PRH	26.2 (150)	8.5 (174)	4.7
NVD < 1/3 DA with VH/PRH	25.6 (39)	4.3 (35)	2.9
NVE $\geq$ 1/2 DA with VH/PRH (in any photographic field)	29.7 (40)	7.2 (41)	3.0

[a]Z value: Observed difference between the proportions of events observed in the untreated and treated groups divided by the standard error of the difference. A Z value of 1.96 is usually associated with a p value significance level of 0.05, a Z value of 2.58 with a p value of 0.01, and a Z value of 3.29 with a p value of 0.001.
[b]NVD, new vessels on or within 1 disc diameter (DD) of the optic disc; NVE, new vessels elsewhere, greater than 1 DD from the optic disc; DA, disc area; HRC, high-risk characteristics; n, number of eyes at risk.

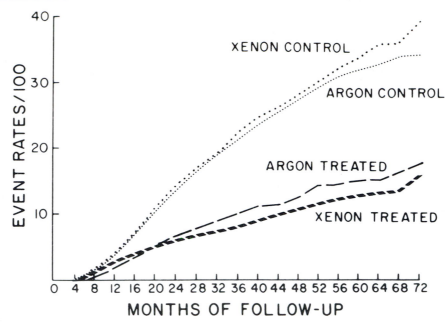

Figure 4–4. Cumulative rates of severe visual loss for argon and xenon groups separately. *(Published courtesy of* Ophthalmology *1981;88:588.)*

effects included a moderate reduction of visual acuity and a constriction of the visual field. It should be noted, however, that the side effects found with xenon treatment were more likely related to the strength of treatment than to the specific light sources used. Xenon complications could most likely be reduced by less intense burns, and intense argon laser burns would probably produce side effects comparable to those found with xenon treatment.

Additional Findings in DRS

The important practical conclusion to draw from these results is that one could support waiting to apply photocoagulation treatment in eyes with NPDR and perhaps also in eyes with PDR but without high-risk characteristics. This would at least defer the risk of undesirable side effects of treatment. Conversely, one should treat eyes with high-risk characteristics as soon as possible to reduce the proven high risk of developing severe visual loss without

TABLE 4–4. DRS: SEVERE VISUAL LOSS IN EYES WITHOUT HRC AT INITIAL VISIT: TREATED VS UNTREATED EYES

| Stage at Initial Visit | % of Eyes at 2 Year Visit with Visual Acuity ≤ 5/200 | | |
	Control (n)	Treated (n)	Z
NVD < 1/3 DA without VH/PRH[a]	10.5 (114)	3.1 (126)	2.4
NVE ≥ 1/2 DA without VH/PRH	6.9 (125)	4.3 (141)	1.0
NVE < 1/2 DA without VH/PRH	6.8 (120)	2.0 (96)	1.8
No new vessels without VH/PRH	3.6 (195)	3.0 (182)	0.4

[a]NVD, new vessels on or within 1 disc diameter (DD) of the optic disc; NVE, new vessels elsewhere, greater than 1 DD from the optic disc; DA, disc area; HRC, high-risk characteristics; n, number of eyes at risk.

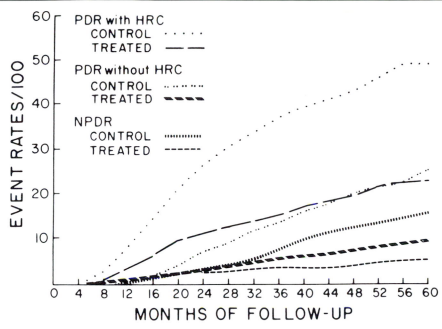

Figure 4–5. Cumulative rates of severe visual loss for eyes classified by presence of proliferative retinopathy (PDR) and high risk characteristics (HRC) in baseline fundus photographs, argon and xenon groups combined. NPDR, nonproliferative diabetic retinopathy. *(Published courtesy of Ophthalmology 1981;88:588.)*

photocoagulation treatment. In eyes with high-risk characteristics, the risk of undesirable side effects is more acceptable because of the poor prognosis without treatment.

The DRS results provide some additional information that might influence whether and when to treat eyes without high-risk characteristics. Photocoagulation treatment was shown to slow the progression of retinopathy. For example, the rate of development of new vessels in eyes without new vessels at entry into the study was reduced by treatment. Similarly, progression to high-risk characteristics or SVL in eyes without high-risk characteristics at entry was slowed, as demonstrated in Table 4–6. The percentage of eyes without high-risk characteristics at the start of the study that at the 1 year visit progressed either to high-risk characteristics, severe visual loss, or ungradable photographs (due to vitreous hemorrhage) was 15.3% in untreated eyes with NPDR at the initial visit. This was reduced to 8.8% by treatment. Similarly 34.6% of untreated eyes with PDR without high-risk characteristics progressed in the same way in 1 year. This was reduced to 14.3% by treatment. Therefore, if the progression to high-risk characteristics in eyes without these high-risk features can be slowed, should one treat such eyes early in the hope that

TABLE 4–5. ESTIMATED PERCENTAGES OF EYES WITH HARMFUL EFFECTS ATTRIBUTABLE TO DRS PHOTOCOAGULATION TREATMENT

	Argon	Xenon
Constriction of visual field (Goldmann IVe4) to an average of		
≤ 45° > 30° per meridian	5%	25%
≤ 30° per meridian	0%	25%
Decrease in visual acuity		
1 line	11%	19%
≥ 2 lines	3%	11%

TABLE 4-6. DRS: RETINOPATHY PROGRESSION SLOWED

| Stage at Initial Visit | % of Eyes at 1-Year Visit with VA < 5/200 or HRC[a] Present, or Photos Ungradable (Presumed Vitreous Hemorrhage) | | |
	Control (n)	Treated (n)	Z
NPDR	15.3 (235)	8.8 (240)	2.2
PDR, HRC absent	34.6 (451)	14.3 (456)	7.1

[a]HRC, high-risk characteristics.

treatment will prevent them from ever developing severe visual loss? Conversely, is it perhaps just as well to withhold treatment in eyes without high-risk characteristics and treat only when and if such poor prognostic signs develop? It is this question that provides the basis for one aspect of the Early Treatment Diabetic Retinopathy Study (ETDRS). Patients with moderate to severe NPDR in both eyes or with PDR but no high-risk characteristics have one eye treated promptly with photocoagulation, and treatment in the opposite eye is deferred unless high-risk characteristics develop.

Severe Fibrous Proliferations

Relatively few eyes in the DRS had severe fibrous proliferation (FP) (less than 10%). There is some concern that photocoagulation might worsen the prognosis in such eyes by inducing shrinkage of fibrous tissue and causing subsequent retinal detachment, particularly in eyes with vitreous hemorrhage, or preexisting vitreoretinal traction, or both. There was evidence in the DRS that xenon-treated eyes with severe FP had an increased incidence of visual loss greater than five lines present at the first visit after treatment and persisting for at least 1 year. Tractional detachment or displacement of the macula was the main mechanism for visual loss.[8] This detrimental treatment side effect was not found in argon-treated eyes. Therefore, one can conclude that the stronger treatment, delivered in xenon-treated eyes, is potentially dangerous in the presence of severe FP, but no evidence of such an effect was found for argon-treated eyes in the DRS, even though complete scatter treatment often was carried out in a single sitting. It would seem wise, however, to apply argon treatment in two or three stages in such eyes. In fact, many surgeons divide panretinal photocoagulation into two sessions (1–2 weeks apart) in all eyes, hoping to prevent tractional complications as well as severe choroidal swelling and serous retinal detachment. Although this is our personal practice, a recent study[9] challenges the necessity of divided treatment with evidence that significant complications are no greater with single than with multiple treatment sessions.

Early vitrectomy in eyes with severe new vessels and fibrous proliferations was tested in the Diabetic Retinopathy Vitrectomy Study (DRVS). Such eyes were randomized to either conventional management (photocoagulation as indicated, but no vitrectomy unless severe persistent vitreous hemorrhage or macular detachment develops) or prompt vitrectomy (with optional previtrectomy photocoagulation). The rationale underlying prompt vitrectomy is that removal of the vitreous eliminates the scaffold for fibrovascular growth, induces regression of existing new vessels, and prevents tractional complications. In this trial, visual acuity of 20/40 or better was observed more frequently during the 4-year follow-up period in the early vitrectomy group. This beneficial effect was striking in the subgroup of eyes with very severe new vessels (at 4 years, 35% of eyes assigned to early vitrectomy had vision at this level compared to 10% of eyes in the deferral group) but became smaller with decreasing severity of new vessels.[10]

Application of DRS Results to Clinical Practice

The following general guidelines for the treatment of eyes with diabetic retinopathy are recommended based on the DRS results. Exception to these general guidelines will be noted also.

Eyes with DRS High-Risk Characteristics

The retinopathy characteristics included in this category and the proportion of eyes that developed severe visual loss without and with treatment are listed in Table 4–3. *Immediate panretinal treatment is recommended.*

Rationale. The overall risk of severe visual loss without treatment (26% at 2 years) and its reduction by treatment (to 11%) outweigh the risk of harmful treatment effects.

Exceptions: (1) The DRS included relatively few eyes with very severe PDR and traction. There is evidence that strong photocoagulation may increase traction on the retina in such eyes, but DRS results support argon scatter photocoagulation in such cases. Consider early vitrectomy in eyes with advanced, active PDR and severe new vessels that have not responded to photocoagulation or cannot be treated adequately because of vitreous hemorrhage. (2) Eyes with severe retinal arteriolar ischemia (Fig. 4–2) also have been reported to develop serious visual loss shortly after extensive scatter treatment, presumably due to photocoagulation-induced macular ischemia.[4] On the other hand, eyes with severe retinal ischemia are also at high risk to develop rubeosis iridis and neovascular glaucoma. Since scatter photocoagulation may inhibit the development of rubeosis iridis, photocoagulation treatment of such eyes would seem desirable. This therapeutic dilemma can be partially resolved by dividing panretinal photocoagulation into several treatments in the hope that this will reduce the impact on the macular circulation. Regardless of the treatment approach, eyes with severe retinal ischemia have a poor prognosis for vision because of the combined effects of proliferative retinopathy, macular ischemia, and neovascular glaucoma.[4]

Eyes Without DRS High-Risk Characteristics but with Severe Nonproliferative or Early Proliferative Retinopathy

The retinopathy characteristics included in this category and the proportion of eyes that developed severe visual loss without and with treatment are listed in Table 4–4. Either of two treatment approaches is reasonable: (1) immediate panretinal treatment or (2) deferral of treatment unless high-risk characteristics develop. Close periodic follow-up is essential to watch for the development of high-risk characteristics.

Rationale. Deferral of treatment postpones, perhaps indefinitely, the risk of harmful treatment effects. If both eyes fall into this category, it is reasonable to treat one eye promptly and defer treatment in the opposite eye unless high-risk characteristics develop.

Exceptions: (1) In eyes with progressive lens changes, prompt treatment is recommended, since further lens opacification might preclude photocoagulation therapy. (2) In female patients who are pregnant and who show substantial retinopathy (severe NPDR or PDR without high-risk characteristics, treatment usually is recommended at least for one eye because of the possibly increased risk of retinopathy progression during pregnancy. (3) Patients with severe NPDR (preproliferative retinopathy) in both eyes who show evidence of progressive diabetic renal failure should probably be photocoagulated promptly because of the poorer visual prognosis when this systemic complication is added. (4) In patients who are unreliable to return for close follow-up care, more prompt treatment may be recommended.

EARLY TREATMENT DIABETIC RETINOPATHY STUDY

Several references to the Early Treatment Diabetic Retinopathy Study (ETDRS) have been made previously in this chapter. This was also a randomized, controlled clinical trial sponsored by the National Eye Institute, and it was a logical outgrowth of the DRS.[11]

Patients eligible for inclusion in the ETDRS were those with diabetic retinopathy in both eyes, either moderate to severe NPDR or PDR without high-risk characteristics. In addition, eyes with macular edema due to diabetic retinopathy were eligible as long as DRS high-risk characteristics were absent. Visual acuity had to be 20/40 or better unless reduced by macular edema (to 20/200 or better). The major questions asked in the ETDRS were as follows.

1. In eyes with diabetic retinopathy without high-risk characteristics, is it better to apply early argon laser photocoagulation (either the full scatter treatment used in the DRS or a milder version) or to defer treatment unless high-risk characteristics develop?

2. In eyes with macular edema due to diabetic retinopathy, is photocoagulation treatment beneficial?

3. Does aspirin treatment slow the progression of diabetic retinopathy?

In order to answer these questions, patients were assigned randomly to aspirin (650 mg once a day) or placebo, and one eye of each patient was assigned randomly to prompt argon laser photocoagulation treatment and the opposite eye was left untreated unless high-risk characteristics developed. The treated eyes were further randomized to mild scatter (400–650 burns) or full scatter (1200–1600 burns). The protocol specified 500 μm burns of moderate intensity scattered from the posterior pole to the equator, spaced evenly one-half to two burn widths apart, as dictated by full or mild scatter assignment. Small patches of flat NVE were treated with confluent burns.

In addition, eyes with macular edema assigned to prompt treatment received focal laser photocoagulation of microaneurysms or other focal leaky lesions in the macular region identified by fluorescein angiography and thought to be contributing to the edema. If the leakage was diffuse, a grid pattern of mild 50 μm to 200 μm diameter burns separated by a burn width were placed in the areas of leakage and in zones of capillary nonperfusion located greater than 500 μm from the center of the macula. Many eyes received focal treatment only, some eyes received a combination of focal and grid treatment, and very few eyes received grid treatment alone. In ETDRS publications, the term "focal photocoagulation" for macular edema is used to include all of these alternatives. In 1985, the ETDRS published convincing evidence of the value of focal photocoagulation for macular edema.[12] In eyes in which the center of the macula was involved by retinal thickening, the 3-year rate of moderate visual loss (defined as a doubling or more of the visual angle, such as a change from 20/20 to 20/40 or worse) was reduced from 33% in untreated eyes to 13% in treated eyes.[13]

Both of the approaches used in the ETDRS to reduce the risk of visual loss from proliferative retinopathy, that is, applying scatter treatment early or withholding it unless high-risk characteristics developed, proved to be effective. The 5-year rate of severe visual loss was 2.5% in eyes assigned to early treatment and 4% in those assigned to deferral.[14] The ETDRS concluded that scatter treatment should not be used in eyes with mild to moderate NPDR but that it should be considered in eyes approaching the high-risk stage and usually should not be delayed when high-risk characteristics are present.

The rationale for studying aspirin in the ETDRS was evidence that abnormal platelet clumping and adhesion are found in some diabetic patients. Since the platelet abnormalities theoretically might contribute to microvascular occlusion in the retina and might be favorably influenced by aspirin therapy, it was hoped that aspirin therapy might reduce retinal ischemia and lessen the stimulus to retinal neovascularization. The ETDRS found no evidence of beneficial or harmful effects of aspirin on the course of diabetic retinopathy and thus no reason to recommend against its use for cardiovascular or other medical indications.[14]

REFERENCES

1. Merin S, Ber I, Ivry M: Retinal ischemia (capillary nonperfusion) and retinal neovascularization in patients with diabetic retinopathy. *Ophthalmologica* 1978; 177:140–145.
2. Kohner EM, Hamilton AM, Joplin GF, Fraser TR: Florid diabetic retinopathy and its response to treatment by photocoagulation or pituitary ablation. *Diabetes* 1976; 25:104–110.
3. Volone JA Jr, McMeel JW: Severe adolescent onset of proliferative diabetic retinopathy: the effect of pituitary ablation. *Arch Ophthalmol* 1978;96:1349–1353.
4. Bresnick GH, De Venecia G, Myers FL, Harris JA, Davis MD: Retinal ischemia in diabetic retinopathy. *Arch Ophthalmol* 1975;93:1300–1310.
5. The Diabetic Retinopathy Study Research Group: Preliminary report on effects of photocoagulation therapy. *Am J Ophthalmol* 1976;81:383–396.
6. The Diabetic Retinopathy Study Research Group: Photocoagulation treatment of proliferative diabetic retinopathy: the second report of Diabetic Retinopathy Study findings. *Ophthalmology* 1978;85:82–106.
7. The Diabetic Retinopathy Study Research Group: Photocoagulation treatment of diabetic retinopathy: clinical application of Diabetic Retinopathy Study (DRS) findings. DRS report number 8. *Ophthalmology* 1981;88:583–600.
8. Diabetic Retinopathy Study Research Group: Photocoagulation treatment of proliferative diabetic retinopathy: relationship of adverse treatment effects to retinopathy severity. DRS report number 5. *Dev Ophthalmol* 1981;2:248–261.
9. Doft BH, Blankenship GW: Single versus multiple treatment sessions of argon laser panretinal photocoagulation for proliferative diabetic retinopathy. *Ophthalmology* 1982;89:772–779.
10. The Diabetic Retinopathy Vitrectomy Study Research Group: Early vitrectomy for severe proliferative diabetic retinopathy in eyes with useful vision. *Ophthalmology* 1988;95:1307–1334.
11. Early Treatment Diabetic Retinopathy Study Research Group: The Early Treatment Diabetic Retinopathy Study: design and baseline patient characteristics. ETDRS report number 7. *Ophthalmology* 1991;98:741–756.
12. Early Treatment Diabetic Retinopathy Study Research Group: Photocoagulation for diabetic macular edema. ETDR Study report number 1. *Arch Ophthalmol* 1985; 103:1796–1806.
13. Early Treatment Diabetic Retinopathy Study Research Group: Photocoagulation for diabetic macular edema. ETDRS report number 4. *Int Ophthalmol Clin* 1987; 27:265–272.
14. Early Treatment Diabetic Retinopathy Study Research Group: *Information for Patients.* Prepared by the Scientific Reporting Section of the National Eye Institute, National Institutes of Health, October 1989.

CHAPTER 5

Proliferative Diabetic Retinopathy

*Mitchell D. Wolf, James C. Folk,
and Michael B. Rivers*

INTRODUCTION

The Diabetic Retinopathy Study (DRS)[1] proved that scatter or panretinal laser photocoagulation (PRP) reduces the risk of visual loss in patients with proliferative diabetic retinopathy (PDR). This chapter describes how to perform panretinal or scatter laser photocoagulation treatment.

DIAGNOSIS

Prelaser Examination

A very important part of the laser treatment is a thorough preoperative evaluation of the patient. Anyone who treats PDR must be facile with the indirect ophthalmoscope. It is the best instrument for examining the retina through vitreous hemorrhage and for studying the complex vitreoretinal abnormalities found in proliferative disease. Clinicians should note areas of extensive background diabetic changes, neovascularization, vitreous hemorrhage, retinal traction, or retinal detachment.

After indirect ophthalmoscopy, the retina must be examined under higher magnification with combinations of the direct ophthalmoscope, the Hruby lens, the 60D or 90D lens, or the plano concave (pancake) contact lens. The

45

direct ophthalmoscope is still very good for detecting neovascularization in the posterior pole and midperiphery. First, the disc should be evaluated, and then the retina should be carefully examined for neovascularization by running along all of the nasal and temporal vascular arcades. The red-free or green light on the direct ophthalmoscope is very useful for detecting neovascularization, which will be highlighted as black vessels over a yellowish background. The direct ophthalmoscope is not particularly good for detection of macular edema because of the lack of stereopsis. The 60D or 90D lens at the slit lamp can be used for the same reasons as the direct ophthalmoscope, that is, for scanning the retina to pick up areas of neovascularization.

The Hruby lens provides good magnification and stereopsis and is useful for evaluating macular edema. It is difficult to use the Hruby to detect neovascularization because of the cumbersome manipulations necessary with the slit lamp and the difficulties in viewing noncentral areas of the retina.

The plano concave (pancake) lens used with the slit lamp is the best device for examining the diabetic retina under high magnification and stereopsis and is especially useful for evaluation of macular edema. Use of this lens, however, necessitates the use of a topical anesthetic and gonioscopic coupling solution, both of which may cause decreased corneal clarity. Therefore, it should not be used before fundus photography.

A practical plan for thoroughly evaluating a diabetic patient would be first to examine the fundi with the indirect ophthalmoscope. This should be followed by a search for neovascularization using either the direct ophthalmoscope or the 60D or 90D lens. Finally, the Hruby lens or pancake contact lens should be used for evaluation of the macula.

PATIENT PREPARATION

The physician should explain to the patient the findings of the ocular examination, the results of the DRS, the laser photocoagulation procedure, the usual side effects after laser treatment, and possible complications. The DRS has proven the value of argon laser photocoagulation in proliferative disease and has shown that it has relatively few side effects and complications. Therefore, the physician should be confident in recommending this therapy, and the discussion with the patient should reflect this confidence. It is not necessary to dwell on all the possible complications, but the patient should be told that after PRP night vision, peripheral vision, and accommodation may be decreased and that the visual acuity may be reduced by one or two lines.[1] Again, these side effects should be balanced against the large benefits from PRP. At this time, the patient should be reminded that laser treatment is not a cure. Many patients are relatively asymptomatic before laser treatment and may develop a vitreous hemorrhage after treatment that they attribute to the laser. The possibility of multiple laser treatments should be stressed before the first treatment. A good prelaser discussion usually will prevent the frustrating situation of a patient refusing further treatment after a postlaser vitreous hemorrhage.

GOALS OF PANRETINAL PHOTOCOAGULATION

The Rodenstock panfunduscopic lens is now popular for panretinal laser treatment. This high plus lens gives an inverted real image of the fundus like that seen with the indirect ophthalmoscope. The lens has a very wide field of view and minifies the fundus structures, allowing for more rapid treatment than when using the pancake and Goldmann three-mirror lenses. The minification of the Rodenstock lens makes it difficult to visualize areas of localized background pathology or areas of neovascularization elsewhere (NVE). These areas of pathology, however, should be noted on the preoperative examination. Because of the minification, laser spot sizes administered with the panfunduscopic lens end up larger than those with the Goldmann lens. For instance, a 350 μm spot with the panfunduscopic lens will cover approximately the same area as a 500 μm spot with the Goldmann lens, and adjustments must be made accordingly. Because of this difference, the following discussion recommends spot sizes for both lens systems.

The goal of panretinal or scatter argon laser treatment is to place 500 μm laser burns using the Goldmann lens systems or 350 μm burns using the Rodenstock lens into the retina one-half to one burn diameter apart from the temporal arcades to the equator. The posterior pole between the temporal arcades and disc is spared, usually comprising an area 2 disc diameters above and below and 2.5 to 3.0 disc diameters temporal to the fovea. If neovascularization of the disc (NVD) is present, the laser spots should come close to the nasal side of the disc approximately one-half burn diameter away. If there is no NVD, the laser burns need not extend any closer than 1 disc diameter nasal to the nervehead. In the DRS, a full argon laser PRP treatment consisted of 800 to 1600 500-μm burns or 500 to 1000 1000-μm burns administered through the pancake or Goldmann three-mirror lens. There is a trend toward a greater number of burns, however, and many ophthalmologists believe that 1600 500-μm burns (350 μm with the Rodenstock lens) is a minimal treatment, and the usual treatment should consist of 2000 or more lesions.

The final area of a laser scar depends on the power used. A higher powered 500-μm burn will result in a greater diameter scar than a light 500-μm burn. Therefore, physicians who administer intense burns will often require fewer spots to cover a given area of retina than will light treaters. The goal of laser treatment should be to induce atrophy of the neovascularization and to apply a good pattern of laser lesions from the posterior pole to the equator. It is inappropriate to consider that a laser treatment should always consist of 1000 or 2000 or 3000 spots. A good average, however for the initial scatter treatment would be approximately 1600 500-μm burns with Goldmann lenses or 350-μm burns with the Rodenstock lens.

The laser spots should be light to medium in intensity, usually a gray to white burn, and be placed one-half to one burn diameter apart (Fig. 5–1). Background abnormalities outside the posterior pole, such as microaneurysms or intraretinal microvascular abnormalities (IRMAs), should be treated directly even if this means disrupting the laser pattern. Neovascularization of the disc should not be treated directly. Focal treatment for highly elevated fronds of NVE usually is unsuccessful. These elevated areas of NVE simply should be surrounded by scatter treatment as usually applied. Areas of NVE that are flat on the retina or minimally elevated are treated with confluent laser burns at the same or perhaps slightly higher intensity than used for the rest of the treatment. Direct occlusion of NVE with small, high-intensity spots is usually unnecessary and may cause rupture of Bruch's membrane and chorioretinal anastomoses.[2] Areas of fibrosis or traction retinal detachment are surrounded but not directly treated because of the danger of causing shrinkage of the scar tissue and increased traction on the retina.

As mentioned, many clinicians now use the Rodenstock lens for routine panretinal treatment. The Rodenstock lens magnifies the entrance pupil, whereas the three-mirror or pancake lens minifies it. Therefore, the Rodenstock lens is especially valuable when treating patients with small pupils. It is also often easier to treat patients with vitreous hemorrhage with the Rodenstock lens than with the Goldmann lens system. Because the pancake Gold-

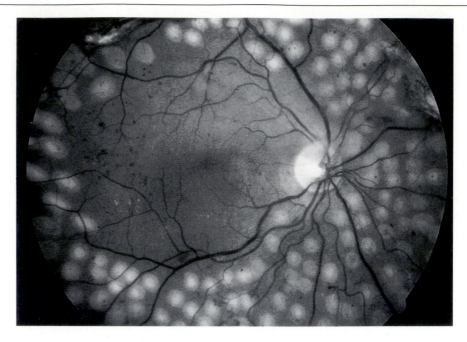

Figure 5–1. Fundus photograph taken immediately after argon panretinal (scatter) photocoagulation. Medium intensity lesions placed about one-half burn diameter apart.

mann lens gives a virtual erect image and the Rodenstock results in an inverted reversed image, clinicians must be very aware of the location of the macula when switching between these lenses so that it is not photocoagulated inadvertently. The relatively new Mainster lens is gaining popularity for scatter treatment of the posterior pole and midperiphery.

There are pros and cons of administering the total scatter treatment in a single session vs in multiple sessions. Doft and Blankenship found that exudative retinal detachments, choroidal detachments, and angle closure occurred more commonly in eyes treated during a single session than in eyes treated in multiple sessions.[3] There were no long-term differences, however, in either beneficial or adverse effects between the single session and the multiple session eyes. The advantages of a single treatment session include convenience to both physician and patient and getting the treatment in before an opacifying vitreous hemorrhage develops. The advantages of multiple treatment sessions are less postoperative ocular pain, fewer postoperative complications, and less need for retrobulbar anesthesia.

The use of single vs multiple treatment sessions should be tailored to the needs of the patient. A single treatment session may be appropriate for a patient who lives far away, has severe neovascularization with traction that is likely to bleed, or absolutely requires retrobulbar anesthesia for any treatment. Multiple treatment sessions may be best if a patient has narrow anterior chamber angles, does not require a retrobulbar injection for 500 to 600 spots during one treatment, or has retinal edema that can increase after scatter laser.

LASER TREATMENT

Patients who are to receive a full scatter treatment of 1200 spots or more in a single session usually require a retrobulbar anesthetic. Multiple session patients who received 500 to 600 spots at each sitting often do not require retrobulbar anesthesia. Young patients, such as juvenile diabetics, require a retrobulbar anesthetic more often than do older patients. The peripheral retina is more sensitive than the posterior pole. The temporal retina is more sensitive than the nasal retina, and areas around the long posterior ciliary nerves are especially sensitive. Usually, a judgment concerning the need for retrobulbar anesthesia can be made before placing the patient at the laser. When in doubt, the treatment can be started, and it will become apparent quickly whether or not a retrobulbar anesthetic is necessary. Lidocaine 2% without epinephrine works well.

If the patient is having mild pain, adjustments in the delivery of the burn can be made to decrease the discomfort. Obviously, larger spot sizes or more intense spots will be more painful than smaller or less intense spots. The shorter the duration of the burn, the less the pain. For instance, a 0.1 sec burn is less painful than a 0.2 sec burn. Although it is nice not to use a retrobulbar anesthetic, ophthalmologists must remember the primary reason for the treatment. If a patient is very uncomfortable and only a few weak spots can be delivered, it is best to interrupt the treatment and administer a retrobulbar anesthetic. Otherwise, there is a great danger of inadequate treatment and poor results.

Typical slit-lamp settings are a 10 × magnification, a 500 μm spot size with Goldmann lenses or 350 μm with the Rodenstock lens, and a 0.1 sec duration (Table 5–1). The power is set on 200 mW and increased in 50 mW increments until there is a light to moderate intensity, gray-white burn. The usual power setting is 250 mW to 450 mW, but more power is necessary in patients with lens opacities, vitreous opacities, or retinal edema. An argon laser with a pure green (514 nm) filter should be used to eliminate the argon blue (488 nm) wavelength. The blue light is absorbed more by a yellow lens nucleus and macular xanthophyll and also is scattered more than the green. The blue light reflected from the aiming beam of an argon blue-green theoretically could also be more harmful to the lens and retina of the treating ophthalmologist than the longer-wavelength pure green light.

TABLE 5–1 Scatter Laser Photocoagulation for Proliferative Diabetic Retinopathy

Spot Size	350 μm Rodenstock
	500 μm Pancake or Goldmann
Duration of Burn	0.1 sec
Initial Power Setting	200mW
Wavelength (nm)	Argon green
Contact Lens	Rodenstock
	Pancake
	Goldmann three-mirror
Anesthesia	Topical or retrobulbar

Goal: Medium-white laser burns should be placed one burn width apart starting outside a 3 disc diameter area superior, inferior, and temporal to the fovea and on nasal side of optic disc. Treatment should extend anterior to the equator. Tailor extent of treatment to severity of retinopathy. Treat flat neovascularization elsewhere with confluent spots. Treat around margins of tractional retinal detachment or elevated fibrovascular stalks. Increase the power in 50 mW increments from the initial setting until the desired intensity is achieved.

The posterior pole is treated first using the pancake lens, the Yannuzzi lens, which is a modification of the pancake lens, or the Rodenstock lens. If the pancake or Yannuzzi lenses are used, the laser burns are first placed nasal to the optic nervehead, which is a relatively safe area until the patient becomes accustomed to the sound, flash, and perhaps mild discomfort of the laser. Once treatment is completed nasal to the disc, it is continued peripheral to the inferior arcade. Care must be taken in patients who do not have a retrobulbar anesthetic when treating directly beneath the macula because a Bell's phenomenon can rotate the macula in front of the laser beam. Next, a double set of spots is placed approximately 2.5 to 3.0 disc diameters temporal to the fovea after a careful check of its position. This double row of spots will serve as a barrier posterior to which treatment should not be placed. The treatment then continues temporally and finally superiorly outside the arcade.

With practice, the pancake or Yannuzzi lens can be used to administer 500 to 600 500-μm spots around the posterior pole. If a patient is being photocoagulated in multiple sessions, this is a good first treatment and usually can be performed without retrobulbar anesthesia. The second treatment session would then consist of administering 500 to 600 500-μm spots over the inferior half of the retina using the equatorial mirror of the Goldmann lens. The third and final treatment session would involve administering 500 to 600 500-μm spots over the superior half of the retina. This method of dividing scatter treatment is convenient because only one lens is required for each of the three treatment sessions (Fig. 5–2).

There are many other ways to divide scatter treatment into multiple sessions, but there is little real difference among methods.[4,5] The posterior pole probably should be demarcated first, however, so a barrier is set up to decrease the chance of macular photocoagulation. Also, because of the danger of vitreous hemorrhage between treatment sessions, the inferior retina should

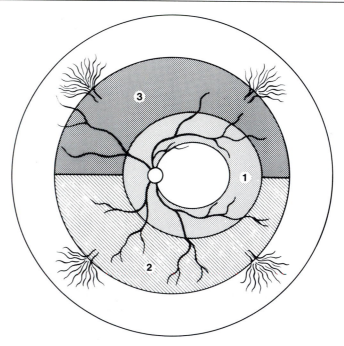

Figure 5–2. Panretinal photocoagulation divided into three treatment sessions using pancake and Goldmann three-mirror lenses. The posterior retina is treated first using the pancake lens (1). Using the equatorial mirror of the Goldmann lens, the inferior midperiphery is treated in the second session (2), and the superior midperiphery is treated in the third (3).

be treated before the superior retina. Single session treated patients are usually given 1200 to 1400 500 μm lesions. The patients are then followed to determine whether this amount of photocoagulation is adequate.

Many clinicians now use the Rodenstock lens for most scatter treatments.[6] Burns administered through the Rodenstock lens are 30% to 40% larger than burns administered through a pancake or Goldmann three-mirror lens. Therefore, a 350 μm burn setting is used with the Rodenstock lens instead of the 500 μm spot size used with the Goldmann lens. The Rodenstock lens can be used to treat in separate sessions as outlined previously. A big advantage of the Rodenstock lens is that it allows for the simultaneous viewing of large portions of the fundus. Clinicians often take advantage of this by treating entire sections of the retina from posterior to anterior during the individual sessions. For example, the clinician could divide the retina into clock hour wedge-shaped sections from 12:00 to 4:00, 4:00 to 8:00, and 8:00 to 12:00. Each of these sections could be treated from posterior to the equator during one of the three treatment sessions (Fig. 5–3).

Usually 1200 to 1800 500 μm burns through the Goldmann lens or 350 μm burns through the Rodenstock lens result in good coverage of the retina and involution of the neovascularization. It is not necessary to routinely place 2000 or more spots in patients with proliferative disease. Patients who receive more extensive treatment often have greater problems with decreased peripheral vision and night vision. Therefore, it is wiser to administer a more moderate number of spots and then follow the patient to determine whether additional photocoagulation is necessary to produce involution of neovascularization. Additional treatment can be added later if necessary. On the other hand, if the patient has severe proliferative retinopathy, the initial laser treatment should be fairly extensive in an attempt to halt rapidly the progression of neovascularization and traction.

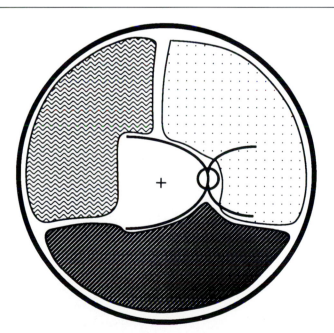

Figure 5–3. PRP divided into three treatment sessions using the Rodenstock lens. This scheme takes advantage of the fact that large sections of retina (such as 12:00–4:00, 4:00–8:00, 8:00–12:00) are seen in one view with the Rodenstock lens. These large wedges are simply filled in from posterior to anterior during a single treatment session. The inferior wedges should be treated first.

POSTTREATMENT CARE

At the end of the laser treatment a cycloplegic drop and an antibiotic steroid ointment are instilled into the conjunctival cul-de-sac, and the eye is patched firmly if the patient has been given a retrobulbar anesthetic. The patient usually is given a short-acting topical cycloplegic drop to be used twice a day and occasionally a topical steroid drop to be used four times a day, both for 1 week. Patients are told to expect mild pain and mild blurriness in vision. They are told to call, however, if they experience severe pain or a severe loss of visual acuity. These severe symptoms could be due to an elevation of intraocular pressure secondary to angle-closure glaucoma.[3,7] Patients who receive treatment all in one session are seen again in 4 to 6 weeks or sooner if they have severe retinopathy. Patients who receive PRP in multiple sessions return weekly for additional treatment.

PATIENT FOLLOW-UP

About 4 to 6 weeks after completion of the laser treatment, the activity of neovascularization should be reassessed, and the completeness of the argon laser coverage should be evaluated by indirect ophthalmoscopy. If the neovascularization is atrophic and there is good coverage, the patient can be discharged and be seen again in 3 months. If the neovascularization is atrophic but the pattern contains large skip areas, the patient should be followed more closely. Neovascularization may recur in these individuals, and they may require additional laser therapy. If neovascularization is still active, additional laser treatment should be administered. Secondary laser treatment should be given to areas of the retina that were skipped or missed during the initial treatment.

The proximity of the laser treatment to the posterior pole also should be checked. Perhaps too wide a berth (5–6 disc diameters) was given around the fovea, and an additional row or two of spots should be placed inside the initial treatment scars. This treatment is especially important if there are areas of ischemic retina in the posterior pole. Signs of ischemic retina include extensive microaneurysms, hemorrhages, intraretinal microvascular abnormalities, and edema. These areas of ischemia are often found temporal to the fovea, and fluorescein angiography is useful in detecting them. Ischemic areas stimulate active neovascularization and should be treated if the neovascularization fails to involute.

Additional laser treatment can be applied in a spot-between-spot fashion. This is especially worthwhile if the pattern of the initial treatment was too loose, meaning the distance between the photocoagulation scars is greater than one-half burn diameter. Finally, additional treatment can be applied peripherally beyond the scars of the initial treatment. Retreatment directly over previous laser scars—in other words, new spots over old spots—does not appear to be beneficial and can result in disruption of Bruch's membrane.

If the neovascularization remains active, argon lesions eventually may be applied confluently well anterior to the equator as well as posteriorly, sparing an area of only approximately 1.5 to 2.0 disc diameters on each side of the fovea. These difficult cases may require as many as 6000 500 μm lesions.

Despite aggressive treatment, some neovascularization may remain open. Occasionally, the active buds of neovascularization will resolve, leaving behind more mature appearing, larger caliber vessels. These vessels are less likely to hemorrhage than are more immature appearing new vessels. Vessels under traction from the vitreous or in fibrovascular membranes may also show incomplete involution. Once the laser treatment is complete, the vessels should be observed. Vitreous surgery should be contemplated if there is severe vitreous hemorrhage or increasing retinal traction. Some physicians advocate peripheral retinal cryoablation after argon laser photocoagulation in recalcitrant cases. Cryopexy seems to work best in eyes with little traction on the retina and persistent neovascularization of the disc. It is important, however, to first treat with the argon laser as much as possible before turning to cryopexy. If progressive vitreoretinal traction occurs, the patient should be considered for vitrectomy rather than have cryopexy.

SPECIAL CASES

Some high-risk patients need special and immediate argon laser treatment. For instance, diabetic patients who have a vitreous hemorrhage that partially obscures the retina have active neovascularization with vitreous traction. They are at high risk for future vitreous hemorrhages and, therefore, should be treated immediately. This is especially true in patients who have hemorrhages confined to the subhyaloid space because often there are large areas of the retina visible that soon will be obscured once the hemorrhage breaks through the hyaloid face into the vitreous cavity (Fig. 5–4). Even partial treatments, such as 400 to 500 lesions applied around areas of hemorrhage, appear to be helpful. These partial treatments may help to turn off neovascularization, decreasing the chance of future hemorrhaging and increasing the chance of additional laser treatment. Too often, these patients are told to return in 6 to 8 weeks when the media clears. Unfortunately, many return with a more severe vitreous hemorrhage than on the first examination.

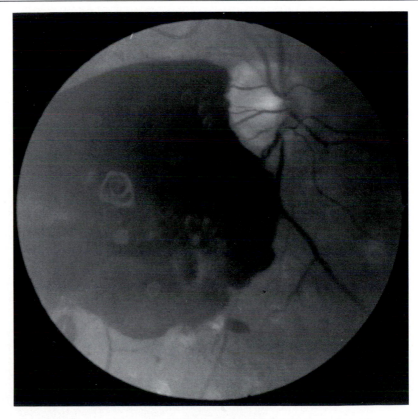

Figure 5–4. Diabetic eye with prehyaloid hemorrhage from neovascularization. Scatter treatment should be placed immediately, before hemorrhage breaks into the vitreous cavity, obscuring the view.

A second special case is the patient who has severe vitreoretinal traction or extramacular tractional retinal detachment. Previously, many ophthalmologists believed that photocoagulation treatment was not indicated in these patients because of a high risk of increasing the traction and causing a retinal detachment. The DRS, however, has shown that argon photocoagulation is both safe and effective for the treatment of these eyes.[8] Areas of epiretinal membrane formation or tractional retinal detachment should be surrounded but not directly photocoagulated (Fig. 5–5).

The third special case is the patient with proliferative retinopathy and a severely edematous retina with extensive background changes. Although these eyes often fare poorly, photocoagulation should be performed. The treatment should be divided into multiple sessions, however, because these eyes are predisposed to serous detachments after photocoagulation. If there is significant macular edema, focal laser treatment should be given before or at the same time of the first scatter treatment.[9]

The final special case is the patient with neovascularization in the anterior chamber angle or neovascular glaucoma. These patients need immediate photocoagulation.[10–12] If the pupil is miotic, a Rodenstock lens will facilitate treatment of the retina. Patients with angle neovascularization have cell and flare in the anterior chamber and need cycloplegics and topical steroids after laser treatment.

KRYPTON LASER

The krypton red laser is described in detail elsewhere[13–15] and appears to be effective in the treatment of diabetic proliferative retinopathy. Red krypton penetrates yellow nuclear sclerotic lenses and vitreous hemorrhage more easily than argon laser. Krypton causes burns in deeper layers of the retina and choroid than argon and thus may result in fewer changes in the internal limiting membrane. This may be an advantage in eyes with vitreoretinal traction

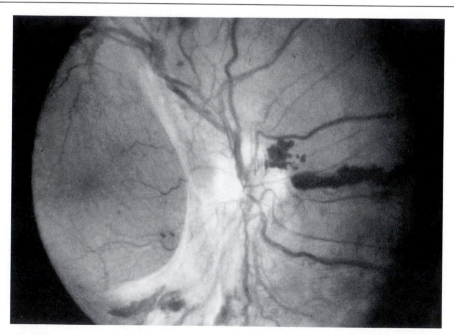

Figure 5–5A. Patient with moderate neovascularization of the disc, fibrosis, and preretinal hemorrhage.

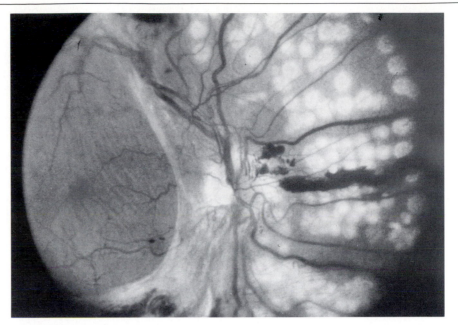

Figure 5–5B. Argon scatter treatment administered around areas of fibrosis.

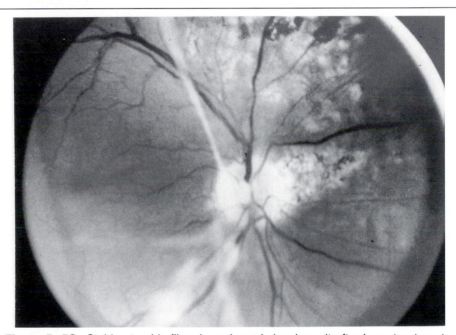

Figure 5–5C. Stable atrophic fibrosis and good visual result after laser treatment.

or macular pucker. The deeper burn of krypton also is a disadvantage because it can cause more postlaser serous choroidal detachments and is more likely to rupture Bruch's membrane and lead to hemorrhages or chorioretinal vascular anastomoses. To reduce the likelihood of disruption of Bruch's membrane, only large spot sizes (350 μm or larger) and long duration burns (at least 0.2 sec) should be used. The end point of a krypton burn is a light grayish white rather than a more white burn as seen with the argon laser. These deeper krypton burns are painful and usually require a retrobulbar anesthetic. Until more work has been done with the krypton laser, the argon green laser is still the treatment of choice in the usual diabetic with proliferative disease.

REFERENCES

1. The Diabetic Retinopathy Study Research Group: Photocoagulation treatment of proliferative diabetic retinopathy: the second report of diabetic retinopathy study findings. *Ophthalmology* 1978;85:82–106.
2. Chandra SR, Bresnick GH, Davis MD, Miller SA, Myers F: Choroidovitreal neovascular ingrowth after photocoagulation for proliferative diabetic retinopathy. *Arch Ophthalmol* 1980;98:1593–1599.
3. Doft BH, Blankenship GW: Single versus multiple treatment sessions of argon laser panretinal photocoagulation for proliferative diabetic retinopathy. *Opthalmology* 1982;89:772–779.
4. Zweng HC, Little HL: *Argon Laser Photocoagulation.* St. Louis: CV Mosby Co; 1977: 180–217.
5. L'Esperance FA, James WA: *Diabetic Retinopathy: Clinical Evaluation and Management.* St. Louis: CV Mosby Co; 1981:146–190.
6. Blankenship GW: Panretinal laser photocoagulation with a wide-angle fundus lens. *Ann Ophthalmol* 1982;14:362–363.
7. Blondeau P, Pavan PR, Phelps CD: Acute pressure elevation following panretinal photocoagulation. *Arch Ophthalmol* 1981;99:1239–1241.
8. Diabetic Retinopathy Study Report No. 5: Photocoagulation treatment of proliferative diabetic retinopathy: relationship of adverse treatment effects to retinopathy severity. *Dev Ophthalmol* 1981;2:248–261.
9. Early Treatment Diabetic Retinopathy Study (EDTRS) Research Group: Effect of scatter photocoagulation therapy on diabetic macular edema. Paper presented by Dr. Robert Murphy at the annual meeting of the American Academy of Ophthalmology, New Orleans, LA, Oct 30, 1989.
10. Little HL, Rosenthal AR, Dellaporta A, Jacobson DR: The effect of panretinal photocoagulation on rubeosis irides. *Am J Ophthalmol* 1976;81:804–809.
11. Jacobson DR, Murphy RP, Rosenthal AR: The treatment of angle neovascularization with panretinal photocoagulation. *Ophthalmology* 1979;86:1270–1275.
12. Pavan PR, Folk JC, Weingeist TA, Hermsen VM, Watzke RC, Montague PR: Diabetic rubeosis and panretinal photocoagulation: a prospective, controlled, masked trial using iris fluorescein angiography. *Arch Ophthalmol* 1983;101:882–884.
13. Schulenburg WE, Hamilton AM, Blach RK: A comparative study of argon laser and krypton laser in the treatment of diabetic optic disc neovascularization. *Br J Ophthalmol* 1979;63:412–417.
14. Singerman LJ, Ferris FL, Mowery RP, Brucker AJ, Murphy RP, Lerner BC, Mincey GJ: Krypton laser for proliferative diabetic retinopathy: the krypton argon regression of neovascularization study. *J Diabetic Comp* 1988;2:189–96.
15. Blankenship GW: Red krypton and blue-green argon panretinal laser photocoagulation for proliferative diabetic retinopathy: a laboratory and clinical comparison. *Trans Am Ophthalmol Soc* 1986;84:967–1003.

CHAPTER 6

Diabetic Macular Edema

Christopher F. Blodi

- Introduction
- Diagnosis
- Laser Treatment
  Preferred Laser Wavelength
  Laser Photocoagulation for Focal Diabetic Macular Edema
  Laser Photocoagulation for Diffuse Diabetic Macular Edema
- References

INTRODUCTION

Many patients with diabetic retinopathy develop macular edema.[1] The prevalence of macular edema is related to the overall severity of the retinopathy and to the duration of diabetes. It is seen more frequently in adult-onset diabetes. Overall, about 10 percent of all diabetics will have retinal thickening within the macula. The fovea will be involved in almost half of these patients.[2]

DIAGNOSIS

Diabetic macular edema can be either focal or diffuse. The pathophysiology of these two variations may be somewhat different. In focal diabetic macular edema, exudate from microaneurysms causes retinal thickening. While this process also occurs in diffuse diabetic macular edema, a significant source of leakage of fluid here is from the entire capillary bed and perhaps even from the choroid across the pigment epithelium.

Decreased perfusion of the capillary bed around the foveal avascular zone can add an ischemic component to the visual loss caused by diabetic macular edema. These eyes generally have a much poorer visual prognosis than eyes with normal perfusion, no matter what treatment modalities are employed.

Fluorescein angiography is an important adjunct in caring for patients with diabetic macular edema. It allows for a more complete understanding of the location and leaking tendencies of microaneurysms and will indicate which patients have diffuse edema. The early phase of the angiogram, especially the laminar venous phase, is especially helpful in analyzing the perfusion of capillaries and the configuration of the foveal avascular zone.

TABLE 6–1. Laser Photocoagulation for Focal Diabetic Macular Edema

Spot Size	50–200 μm
Duration of Burn	0.1 sec
Initial Power Setting	100 mW
Wavelength	Argon green
Contact Lens	Goldmann or Yanuzzi
Anesthesia	Topical

Goal: The microaneurysms are treated with 50–100 μm spot size. Some larger microaneurysms will change color to white or dark when directly treated, but many microaneurysms will not. Initial laser spots will whiten the outer retina and pigment epithelium under the microaneurysms. Then three to four repeat applications of laser energy to the microaneurysm can be applied, using the deeper initial burn to protect the pigment epithelium and to help obtain more energy uptake at the microaneurysm. Often, a smaller spot size than the initial application is used on the repeat applications. Areas of nonperfusion outside the fovea can be treated with a grid array of laser spots using 100 μm spot size and 1 burn width apart. All areas of affected retina (microaneurysms and areas of nonperfusion) at least 500 μm beyond the center of the macula should be treated.

The power can be increased in 50 mW increments from the initial setting until the desired intensity is achieved. If inadequate burns are obtained at 500 mW, consideration can be given to increasing the duration to 0.2 sec. If this is still inadequate, consideration can be given to shifting to krypton red or dye yellow laser photocoagulation, also at 0.2 sec.

It is important to remember to check for proliferative diabetic retinopathy when examining patients for diabetic macular edema. Subtle proliferative changes may occur during the period when the ophthalmologist is most concerned with carefully studying the macula. Because of the treatment implications of proliferative diabetic retinopathy and because of certain treatment strategies for patients with both proliferative diabetic retinopathy and diabetic macular edema, it is important to check always for the presence of proliferative retinopathy.

Recent work has shown the possible efficacy of early mild or full "scatter" (panretinal) photocoagulation for severe nonproliferative diabetic retinopathy or early proliferative diabetic retinopathy. If a decision is made to perform laser photocoagulation for this amount of diabetic retinopathy, careful attention should be paid to the presence or absence of diabetic macular edema. If diabetic macular edema is present, focal laser photocoagulation probably should be performed first. There may be a risk of exacerbating diabetic macular edema in these patients after panretinal photocoagulation is performed.

LASER TREATMENT

Preferred Laser Wavelength

The Early Treatment Diabetic Retinopathy Study (ETDRS)[3,4] used both argon blue-green and green wavelength laser photocoagulation. However, it is clear that the blue wavelength adds little to the treatment effect. Additionally, absorption of blue light by xanthochrome lens pigment and xanthophyll in the macula makes this wavelength undesirable. Argon green is, therefore, the best choice for treating diabetic macular edema.

Laser Photocoagulation for Focal Diabetic Macular Edema

The ETDRS clearly showed the efficacy of focal laser treatment for diabetic macular edema that was "clinically significant." This was defined as retinal thickening within 500 μm of the center of the macula or hard exudate within 500 μm of the center of the macula, with associated thickening of adjacent retina, or an area of thickening at least 1 disc area in size that was within 1 disc diameter (DD) of the center of the macula. Laser treatment was especially useful in reducing the rate of visual loss when the center of the macula was involved with retinal thickening.

Guidelines for treating focal diabetic macular edema include

1. Visual acuity of 20/20 to 20/200

2. "Clinically significant" macular edema, as described by the ETDRS

3. Recent fluorescein angiogram to identify leaking microaneurysms and areas of nonperfusion

Laser photocoagulation is administered as outlined in Table 6–1 (Fig. 6–1). Topical anesthesia usually is adequate and enables one to treat both eyes at a single sitting, if necessary. Retrobulbar anesthesia can be used if excessive patient eye movement is a problem.

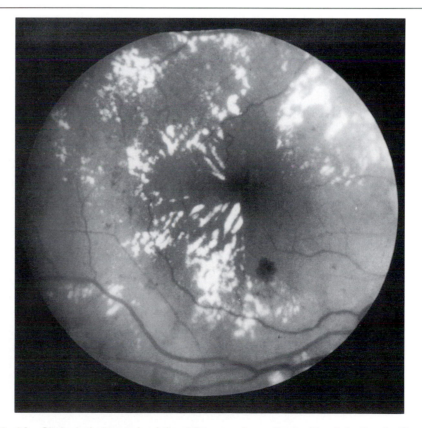

Figure 6–1A. Clinical photograph of the right eye of a patient with clinically significant diabetic macular edema.

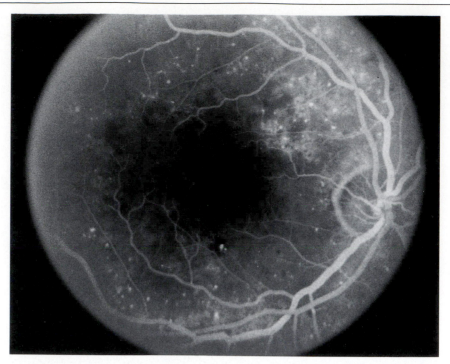

Figure 6–1B. Mid-phase fluorescein angiogram demonstrating punctate areas of hyperfluorescence consistent with microaneurysms.

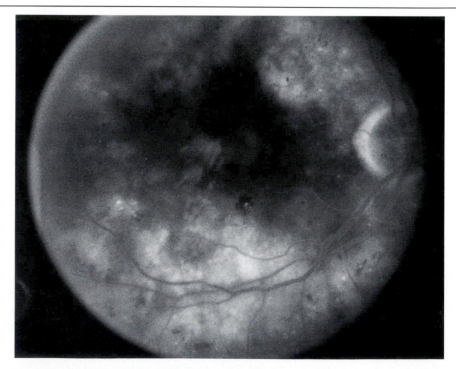

Figure 6–1C. Late phase fluorescein angiogram demonstrating progressive fluorescein leakage.

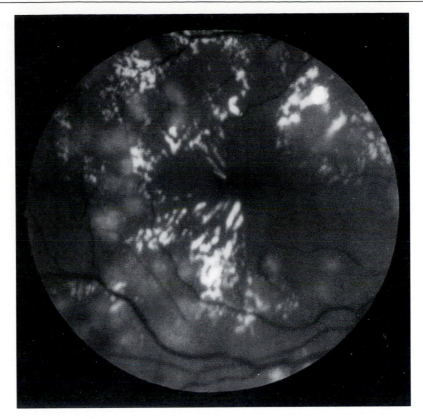

Figure 6–1D. Fundus photograph immediately after argon green focal laser treatment, showing the light and moderate laser burns directed toward leaking microaneurysms.

Patients usually are seen in a follow-up visit 2 to 4 months after treatment. Resolution of edema may be quite slow. Generally, retreatment is not indicated any earlier than 3 to 4 months. Repeat fluorescein angiograms often are helpful to detect new or persistent areas of leaking microaneurysms or untreated areas of nonperfusion. Retreatment often is necessary if there is worsening of the edema or if persistent leakage from previously treated microaneurysms is present. The same treatment strategies used at the initial session (Table 6–1) are employed. Follow-up visits after stability has been achieved are required at 4- to 6-month intervals. This enables the physician to monitor for exacerbations of the macular edema as well as for signs of proliferative retinopathy.

Laser Photocoagulation for Diffuse Diabetic Macular Edema

Diffuse macular edema generally is difficult to treat satisfactorily. Patients often have a symmetrical maculopathy and frequently have systemic conditions that exacerbate their diffuse edema. Attention to treating cardiovascular, renal, hypertensive, and triglyceride abnormalities may facilitate resolution of diffuse macular edema.

Fluorescein angiography is useful in identifying areas of focal leakage that can be treated specifically and in identifying areas of nonperfusion that may be treated.

Guidelines for treating diffuse diabetic macular edema include[5]

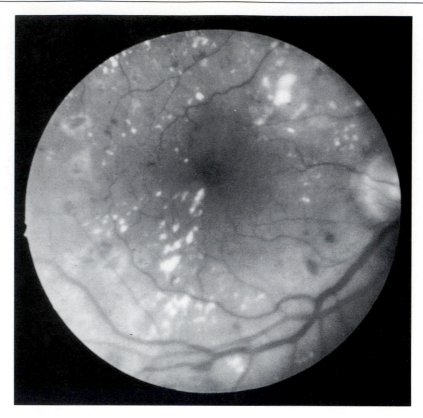

Figure 6–1E. Fundus photograph 6 months after laser treatment. Note the laser scars and significant resolution of the intraretinal lipid exudate.

TABLE 6–2. Laser Photocoagulation for Diffuse Diabetic Macular Edema

Spot Size	100–200 μm
Duration of Burn	0.1 sec
Initial Power Setting	100 mW
Wavelength	Argon green
Contact Lens	Goldmann or Yanuzzi
Anesthesia	Topical

Goal: Medium-white burns are placed in a grid configuration, sparing a central radius 500 μm from fixation. The innermost burns are usually 100 μm in size, and the more peripheral ones are 100–200 μm in size. Burns are placed with 1 burn width spacing. Treatment usually is extended as far as is necessary, using the fluorescein angiogram as a guide (often to the major vascular arcade). Power is increased in 50 mW increments as necessary. Microaneurysms should be specifically treated, as described in Table 6–1.

1. Visual acuity of 20/20 to 20/200

2. Diffuse retinal thickening that is "clinically significant"

3. Recent fluorescein angiographic documentation

Laser photocoagulation is administered as in Table 6–2 (Fig. 6–2). Topical anesthesia is almost always adequate and allows treatment of both eyes, if desired, at one setting. Retrobulbar anesthesia can be used if excessive patient eye movement is present.

Patients usually are reevaluated 3 to 4 months after treatment. Persistent diffuse edema often is present, and retreatment may still be beneficial. Retreatment should consist of placing additional laser burns between preexisting spots and tightening the grid pattern to within 200 μm of fixation. Follow-up visits every 4 to 6 months are necessary to monitor for stability of the treatment and to look for proliferative diabetic retinopathy.

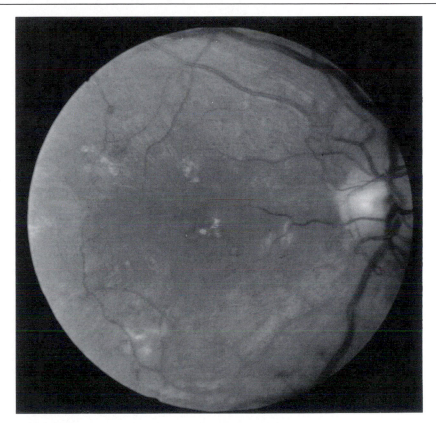

Figure 6–2A. Fundus photograph of an 18-year-old diabetic with proliferative diabetic retinopathy and diffuse macular edema. Note the central macular cyst.

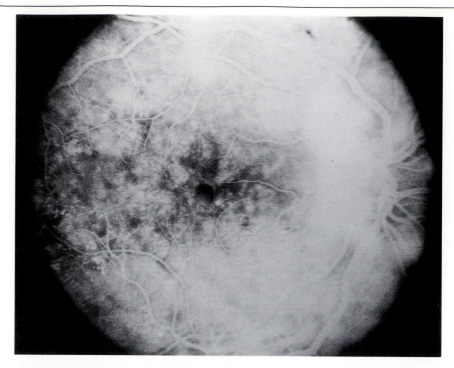

Figure 6–2B. Midphase fluorescein angiogram demonstrating the diffuse fluorescein leakage in the macula. Note the intense hyperfluorescence from the disc neovascularization.

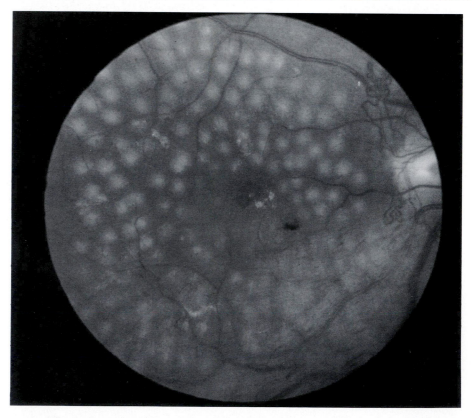

Figure 6–2C. Immediately after argon green grid laser treatment to the areas of retinal thickening using 100 μm spots. The burns were spaced approximately 1 burn width apart.

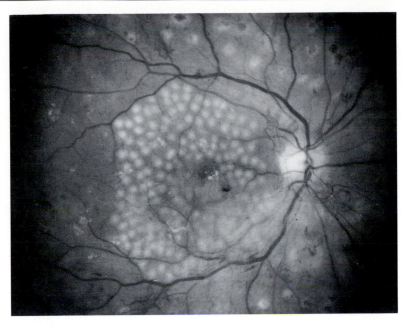

Figure 6–2D. A 60 degree photograph after grid laser photocoagulation.

REFERENCES

1. Bresnick GH: Background diabetic retinopathy. In: Ryan SJ, ed. *Retina*. St. Louis, MO: CV Mosby Co; 1989;2:327–366.
2. Klein R, Klein BEK, Moss SE, Davis MD, DeMets DL: The Wisconsin epidemiologic study of diabetic retinopathy: IV. Diabetic macular edema. *Ophthalmology* 1984;91:1464–1474.
3. Early Treatment Diabetic Retinopathy Study Research Group: Photocoagulation for diabetic macular edema: Early Treatment Diabetic Retinopathy Study report No. 1. *Arch Ophthalmol* 1985;103:1796–1806.
4. Early Treatment Diabetic Retinopathy Study Research Group: Treatment techniques and clinical guidelines for photocoagulation of diabetic macular edema: Early Treatment Diabetic Retinopathy Study report No. 2. *Ophthalmology* 1987;94:761–774.
5. Olk RJ: Modified grid argon (blue-green) laser photocoagulation for diffuse diabetic macular edema. *Ophthalmology* 1986;93:938–950.

CHAPTER 7

Branch Retinal Vein Occlusion

Scott R. Sneed

INTRODUCTION

Branch retinal vein occlusion (BRVO) is one of the most common retinal vascular disorders seen by the ophthalmologist, and it often is associated with systemic hypertension. Branch retinal vein occlusions occur at arterial venous crossing sites. Temporal BRVOs most frequently come to the attention of the ophthalmologist because of associated macular edema.

DIAGNOSIS

Ophthalmoscopically, acute BRVO is characterized by segmental intraretinal or subretinal hemorrhage, retinal edema, and occasionally cotton-wool spots. The location of the retinal pathologic condition in BRVO is determined by that area of the retina that is drained by the occluded branch retinal vein. As the retinal hemorrhages resolve, chronic changes of BRVO may occur, including chronic macular edema and retinal lipid exudate, dilated collateral vessels that may develop along the horizontal raphe, capillary nonperfusion, microaneurysm formation, venous sheathing, epiretinal membrane formation, macular hole formation, retinal or disc neovascularization, vitreous hemorrhage, and traction or rhegmatogenous retinal detachment, or both.

Acutely, fluorescein angiography may be difficult to interpret because of fluorescein blockage by the intraretinal hemorrhage. Fluorescein angiography, therefore, often is not particularly useful in acute BRVO. When most of the intraretinal hemorrhage has cleared, fluorescein angiography may reveal capillary nonperfusion, collateral vessel formation, other retinal vascular abnormalities, macular edema, and retinal neovascularization.

In eyes with a temporal BRVO, macular edema is almost always present.[1] Macular edema spontaneously resolves without treatment in 40 to 50 percent of these eyes over 4 to 6 months.[1,2] Macular edema may develop also in eyes with a macular BRVO. These eyes should be managed in the same manner as temporal BRVOs.

Retinal or disc neovascularization may develop several months after the onset of the BRVO. Neovascularization is almost always accompanied by large areas of capillary nonperfusion (retinal ischemia). Retinal neovascularization develops in approximately 25% of eyes with a temporal BRVO. Neovascularization may lead to vitreous hemorrhage, traction, rhegmatogenous retinal detachment or all of these. Tortuous collateral vessels may resemble neovascularization ophthalmoscopically. Fluorescein angiography is useful in differentiating between these two entities. Neovascularization tends to leak more fluorescein than do collateral vessels.

LASER TREATMENT

Preferred Laser Wavelength

The Branch Vein Occlusion Study Group found argon laser to be effective in treating macular edema and preretinal neovascularization complicating BRVO.[3,4] Therefore, argon green is probably the wavelength of choice in the routine treatment of macular edema and preretinal neovascularization in these eyes. Argon blue-green can also be used, but the blue wavelength is absorbed by the xanthochrome lens pigments and the macular xanthophyll.

Adequate argon laser photocoagulation may be prevented by vitreous hemorrhage or cataract. In these eyes, krypton red laser photocoagulation has proven effective in the treatment of macular edema and preretinal neovascularization associated with BRVO.[5]

Laser Photocoagulation of Macular Edema Associated with Branch Retinal Vein Occlusion

Chronic macular edema may result in persistent visual loss in patients with BRVO. The BVO Study concluded that grid argon laser photocoagulation improves the visual outcome in eyes with BRVO and vision of 20/40 or worse due to macular edema.[3] The following guidelines for laser treatment of macular edema in BRVO are adapted from the recommendations made by the BVO Study Group.

1. BRVO at least 3 months old (segmental retinal hemorrhages probably signify a recent vein occlusion)

2. Visual acuity of 20/40 or worse

3. Fluorescein angiographic evidence of macular edema involving the fovea

4. Fluorescein angiographic documentation less than 1 month old

5. Absence of hemorrhage in the fovea

6. Clearing of retinal hemorrhages to allow accurate interpretation of the fluorescein angiogram and safe laser photocoagulation

7. Absence of foveal ischemia

Laser photocoagulation (Fig. 7–1) is administered as outlined in Table 7–1. Although topical anesthesia usually is adequate, excessive patient eye movement may require a retrobulbar anesthetic. Argon green is the preferred wavelength, although krypton red may be used in the presence of cataract or vitreous hemorrhage. Eyes treated with krypton red may require retrobulbar anesthesia to avoid discomfort. Ruptures of Bruch's membrane can be avoided by increasing the duration of krypton red laser burns to 0.2 sec.

Patients should be seen at 4-month intervals after laser treatment. If persistent macular edema is observed on clinical examination and if visual loss persists, fluorescein angiography should be repeated. Areas of persistent leakage can be retreated with laser photocoagulation. Several retreatments may be necessary to control the macular edema (four eyes in the BVO Study were treated five times). Follow-up visits every 6 to 12 months are reasonable once the macular edema has stabilized, unless the patient notes metamorphopsia or decreased vision.

Laser Photocoagulation for Preretinal Neovascularization Associated with Branch Retinal Vein Occlusion

Results from the Branch Vein Occlusion Study suggest that laser photocoagulation be administered to eyes with a BRVO associated with retinal neovascularization. Results from this study also suggest that there may be no advantage in treating eyes with a BRVO to prevent the development of neovascularization.[4]

Trempe et al. found a high risk of preretinal neovascularization and vitreous hemorrhage in eyes with BRVO and no posterior vitreous detachment-

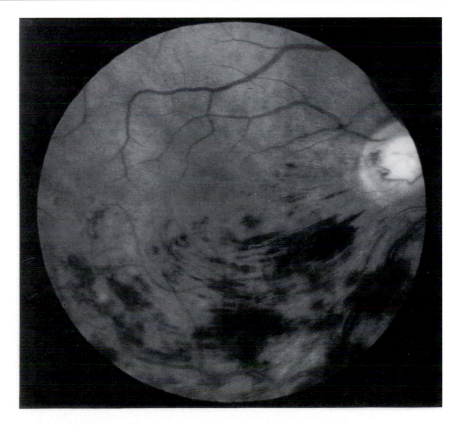

Figure 7–1A. Acute inferotemporal branch retinal vein occlusion of the right eye.

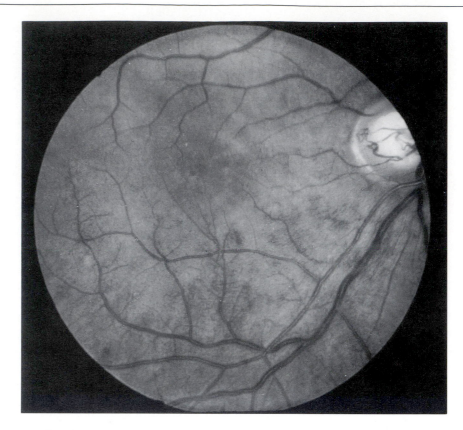

Figure 7–1B. Fundus photograph 4 months after initial presentation. Note resolution of the intraretinal hemorrhages.

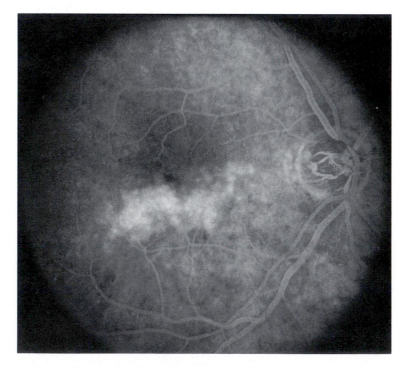

Figure 7–1C. Fluorescein angiogram demonstrating localized macular edema.

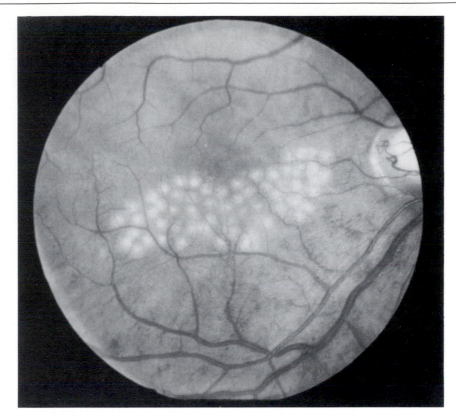

Figure 7–1D. Photograph immediately after argon green laser treatment with sparing of the foveal avascular zone. Laser was administered to the areas of fluorescein leakage.

(PVD) or partial PVD. No patient in their series developed preretinal neovascularization if a complete PVD was present.[6] Based on these results, observation without laser treatment may be warranted in eyes with preretinal neovascularization and a complete PVD. If a definite complete PVD is not observed or if a partial PVD or no PVD is present, laser photocoagulation is warranted in eyes with preretinal neovascularization. Any eye with vitreous hemorrhage and preretinal neovascularization probably should receive laser photocoagulation. Fluorescein angiography performed after clearing of the retinal hemorrhages is useful in determining areas of capillary nonperfusion.

Laser photocoagulation is administered as outlined in Table 7–2. Although topical anesthesia usually is adequate, some patients may require retrobulbar anesthesia to avoid discomfort from the laser treatment. Argon green is preferred in most eyes with preretinal neovascularization. If vitreous hemorrhage or cataract is present, however, the krypton red laser may be necessary for adequate photocoagulation. Eyes treated with krypton red may require retrobulbar anesthesia. Burn duration in krypton red treatment should range from 0.2 to 0.5 sec to avoid rupture of Bruch's membrane. Laser photocoagulation is administered to that portion of the fundus affected by the BRVO (Fig. 7–2). The surrounding normal and unaffected retina should not be treated.

Patients are seen 4 to 6 weeks after laser treatment. If regression of the preretinal neovascularization is noted, further observation is suggested. If the preretinal neovascularization shows no sign of regression or if vitreous hemorrhage occurs 4 to 6 weeks after treatment, additional laser photocoagulation is administered. After regression of the preretinal neovascularization, 6- to 12-month follow-up is reasonable unless the patient notes decreased vision or new floaters.

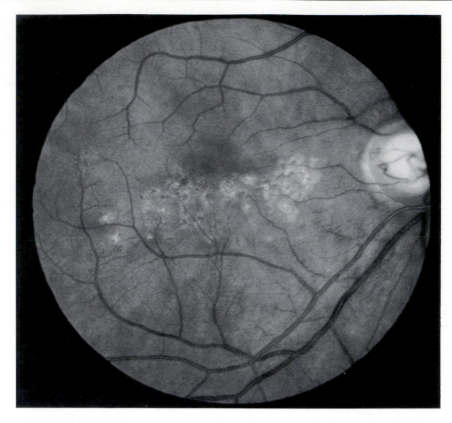

Figure 7–1E. Photograph 4 months after grid laser treatment with no residual macular edema.

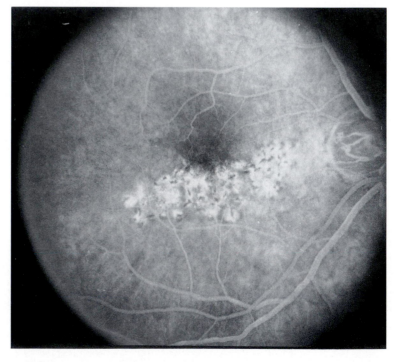

Figure 7–1F. Fluorescein angiogram 4 months after laser treatment showing no evidence of residual macular edema.

TABLE 7–1. Laser Photocoagulation for Macular Edema Associated with Branch Retinal Vein Occlusion

Spot Size	100–200 μm
Duration of Burn	0.1 sec
Initial Power Setting	150 mW
Wavelength	Argon green
Contact Lens	Goldmann or Yanuzzi
Anesthesia	Topical

Goal: Medium-white laser burns spaced 1 burn width apart to the area of fluorescein leakage, no closer to the fovea than the edge of foveal avascular zone. Avoid treating collateral vessels, and avoid treating within the foveal avascular zone. Two to three rows of 100 μm spots are administered along the edge of the foveal avascular zone, and 200 μm spots are used in the more peripheral macula within the major vascular arcade.

Note: Increase the power in 50 mW increments from the initial setting until the desired intensity is achieved. In very edematous retina, burns may be inadequate at 500 mW. If so, turn power to 250 mW and increase the duration to 0.2 sec. Gradually increase power by 50 mW increments until desired intensity is achieved.

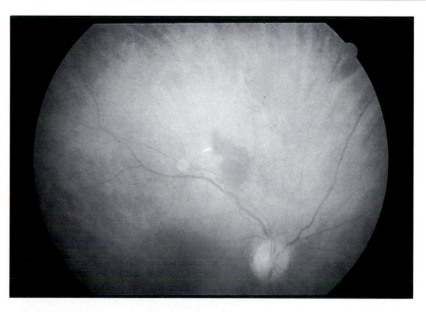

Figure 7–2A. Superotemporal branch retinal vein occlusion. Note the retinal vascular changes and the preretinal hemorrhage from neovascularization elsewhere limited to the superotemporal quadrant.

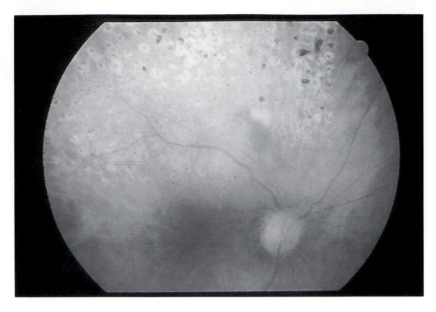

Figure 7–2B. One year after sector laser photocoagulation to the portion of the fundus affected by the vein occlusion. Persistent preretinal hemorrhage and neovascularization persist and warrant further laser treatment.

TABLE 7–2. Laser Photocoagulation for Neovascularization Associated with Branch Retinal Vein Occlusion

Spot Size	200–500 μm
Duration of Burn	0.1 sec
Initial Power Setting	200 mW
Wavelength	Argon green
Contact Lens	Rodenstock
Anesthesia	Topical

Goal: Medium-white laser burns spaced 1 burn width apart to the areas of ischemia noted clinically and angiographically, sparing the area within the temporal vascular arcade. Flat neovascularization outside the macula and disc may be treated with confluent laser. Elevated neovascularization and areas of vitreoretinal traction should be surrounded by laser when outside the macula but should not be photocoagulated directly.

Note: Increase the power in 50 mW increments from the initial setting until the desired burn intensity is achieved. More power is necessary for larger spot sizes. If the burn is inadequate at 700 mW, decrease the power to 400 mW and increase the duration of the burn to 0.2 sec. Again, increase power in 50 mW increments until the desired burn intensity is achieved. Retrobulbar anesthesia may be necessary for burns of greater than or equal to 0.2 sec.

REFERENCES

1. Michels RG, Gass JDM: The natural course of retinal branch vein obstruction. *Trans Am Acad Ophthalmol Otolaryngol* 1974;78:166–177.
2. Gutman FA, Zegarra H: The natural course of temporal retinal branch vein occlusion. *Trans Am Acad Ophthalmol Otolaryngol* 1974;78:178–192.
3. Branch Vein Occlusion Study Group: Argon laser photocoagulation for macular edema in branch vein occlusion. *Am J Ophthalmol* 1984;98:271–282.
4. Branch Vein Occlusion Study Group: Argon laser scatter photocoagulation for prevention of neovascularization and vitreous hemorrhage in branch vein occlusion: a randomized clinical trial. *Arch Ophthalmol* 1986;104:34–41.
5. Roseman RL, Olk RJ: Krypton red laser photocoagulation for branch retinal vein occlusion. *Ophthalmology* 1987;94:1120–1125.
6. Trempe CL, Takahaski M, Topilow HW: Vitreous changes in retinal branch vein occlusion. *Ophthalmology* 1981;88:681–687.

CHAPTER 8

Central Serous Retinopathy

Robert C. Watzke

■ **Introduction**
■ **Diagnosis**
■ **Indications**
■ **Laser Treatment**
    Severe Forms of Central Serous Choroidopathy
■ **References**

INTRODUCTION

Central serous retinopathy is an idiopathic disease that tends to affect one or both eyes of otherwise healthy, young and middle-aged patients. Patients may have symptoms of metamorphopsia, micropsia, decreased vision, or a relative scotoma.

DIAGNOSIS

Clinically, central serous retinopathy is characterized by a neurosensory retinal detachment, usually located in the macula. Fluorescein angiography demonstrates one or more focal leaking areas at the level of the retinal pigment epithelium (RPE), some of which may attain the characteristic smokestack-like appearance.

Three well-planned clinical trials have proven that this disease can be shortened by laser photocoagulation to the area of active fluorescein leakage.[1–3] Laser photocoagulation under the serous detachment, but away from the point of leakage, is useless.[3,4] It also has been proven that shortening the duration of the disease does not improve the final visual acuity.[1–5] Finally, subretinal neovascular membranes may develop from a laser burn, causing serious and permanent loss of central vision.[6]

INDICATIONS

Therefore, treatment of the average case of central serous retinopathy whose duration is less than 6 months is not recommended. About 80 percent of patients will have recovered spontaneously by that time. Most patients will prefer to wait for spontaneous recovery if they are informed of the favorable

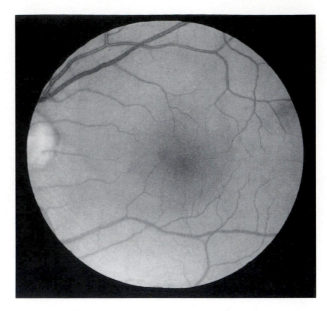

Figure 8–1A. Fundus photograph of the left eye of a 48-year-old white male with central serous retinopathy. Note the macular subretinal fluid involving the fovea.

prognosis and possible complications. There are, of course, exceptional patients whose vocational needs will require early treatment. The risks vs benefits should be explained to all patients, and treatment should not be advised except for compelling reasons.

LASER TREATMENT

If treatment is elected, it consists of placement of moderate intensity argon laser burns (Fig. 8–1) over all sites of active leakage clustered so as to cover the entire leak (Table 8–1). In order to avoid fracture of Bruch's membrane and posttreatment subretinal neovascular membranes, burns should be no less than 100 μm in size and should be just intense enough to produce only a moderate whitening of the RPE. The duration is usually 0.1 sec. Treatment is guided by reference to an early frame of a recent angiogram. The operator must be sure to cover all areas of active leakage. Laser photocoagulation can

TABLE 8–1. Laser Photocoagulation of Central Serous Choroidopathy	
Spot Size	100–200 μm
Duration of Burn	0.1 sec
Initial Power Setting	75 mW
Wavelength	Argon green, krypton red
Contact Lens	Goldmann
Anesthesia	Topical

Goal: Minimal whitening of the retinal pigment epithelium clustered to cover all areas of active leakage, as noted in a recent angiogram.

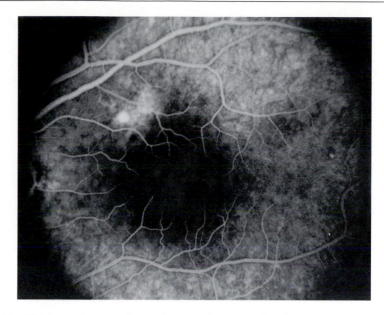

Figure 8–1B. Midphase fluorescein angiogram demonstrating the punctate area of fluorescein leakage in the superonasal macula.

be done under the macular papular bundle without producing a central scotoma. Treatment should not be performed within the fovea, since patients will notice a postoperative scotoma.

All controlled trials have used either ruby laser or argon blue-green as the treatment wavelength. It seems reasonable that argon green would be the wavelength of choice, since the goal of treatment is to produce burns in the RPE and outer retina. One early trial confirmed the efficacy of ruby laser (694 nm) in the treatment of central serous choroidopathy. This would indicate

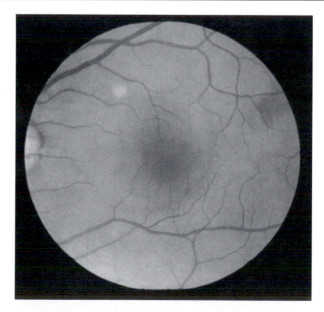

Figure 8–1C. Fundus photograph immediately after light argon green laser photocoagulation.

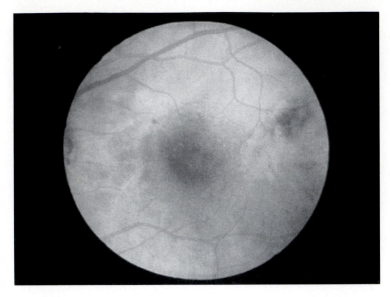

Figure 8–1D. Fundus photograph 6 months after successful laser treatment. Note resolution of the subretinal fluid.

that krypton laser (647 nm) would also be effective. A recent study suggested this, although the study was retrospective and uncontrolled.[7]

Severe Forms of Central Serous Choroidopathy

There is a special form of central serous choroidopathy that consists of prolonged serous detachment with multiple and recurrent leaks.[8–11] This indolent serous detachment causes scarring and proliferation of the RPE to a striking degree, which is easily recognized on fluorescein angiography but is less obvious on clinical examination. Frequently, the RPE is scarred in a vertically linear fashion because subretinal fluid has pooled from the posterior pole into the inferior fundus. Active leaks are hard to recognize against the background of transmission defects caused by RPE scarring. Consequently, these cases are difficult to treat, and recurrence is the rule.

REFERENCES

1. Watzke RC, Burton TC, Leaverton PE: Ruby laser photocoagulation therapy of central serous retinopathy; Part I: A controlled clinical study; Part II: Factors affecting prognosis. *Trans Am Acad Ophthalmol Otolaryngol* 1974;78:OP-205–OP-211.
2. Leaver P, Williams C: Argon laser photocoagulation in the treatment of central serous retinopathy. *Br J Ophthalmol* 1979;63:674–677.
3. Robertson DM, Ilstrup D: Direct, indirect, and sham laser photocoagulation in the management of central serous chorioretinopathy. *Am J Ophthalmol* 1983;95: 457–466.
4. Watzke RC, Burton TC, Woolson RF: Direct and indirect laser photocoagulation of central serous choroidopathy. *Am J Ophthalmol* 1979;88:914–918.
5. Ficker L, Vafidis G, While A, Leaver P: Long-term follow-up of a prospective trial of argon laser photocoagulation in the treatment of central serous retinopathy. *Br J Ophthalmol* 1988;72:829–834.
6. Schatz H, Yannuzzi LA, Gitter HA: Subretinal neovascularization following argon laser photocoagulation treatment for central serous chorioretinopathy: complication or misdiagnosis? *Trans Am Acad Ophthalmol Otolaryngol* 1977;83:OP-893–OP-906.

7. Novak MA, Singerman LJ, Rice TA: Krypton and argon laser photocoagulation for central serous chorioretinopathy. *Retina* 1987;7:162–169.
8. Zweng HC: Diffuse retinal pigment epitheliopathy. In: Zweng HC, Little HA, eds. *Argon Laser Photocoagulation*. St. Louis, MO: CV Mosby; 1977:117–126.
9. Verdaquer J, Ibanez S, LeClerq NL: Unusual and severe forms of central serous chorioretinopathy. In: Ryan SJ, Dawson AK, Little HL, eds. *Retinal Diseases*. Orlando, FL: Grune & Stratton; 1985:151–154.
10. Jalkh A, Jabbour N, Avila MP, Trempe CL, Schepens CL: Retinal pigment epithelial decompensation; Part I: Clinical features and natural course; Part II: Laser treatment. *Ophthalmology* 1984;91:1544–1553.
11. Yannuzzi L, Shakin J, Fisher YL, Altomonte MA: Peripheral retinal detachments and retinal pigment epithelial atrophic tracts secondary to central serous choroidopathy. *Ophthalmology* 1984;91:1554–1572.

CHAPTER 9

Choroidal Neovascular Membranes in Aging Macular Degeneration and the Presumed Ocular Histoplasmosis Syndrome

Warren M. Sobol, James C. Folk, and Mitchell D. Wolf

INTRODUCTION

Aging macular degeneration (AMD) is the leading cause of new cases of legal blindness in people 65 or older in the United States. Most patients who become legally blind do so from complications of choroidal neovascular membranes. Visual loss in the presumed ocular histoplasmosis syndrome (POHS) also is caused by choroidal neovascular membranes growing in and around old histoplasmosis scars. POHS affects mainly patients age 25 through 50 who live in the eastern half of the midwestern United States.

The Macular Photocoagulation Study (MPS)[1–4] is a multicentered, randomized trial designed to evaluate laser photocoagulation in patients with choroidal neovascular membranes secondary to AMD or POHS. In two separate trials, the MPS showed that argon blue-green laser treatment reduced visual loss in patients with choroidal neovascular membranes 200 μm or more from the center of the foveal avascular zone due to either AMD or POHS. In two subsequent trials, the MPS showed that krypton red laser photocoagulation of choroidal neovascular membranes within 200 μm of the center of the fovea, but not beneath the center, also reduced visual loss in patients with AMD or POHS.[3,4] Currently, an MPS trial is evaluating the efficacy of laser photocoagulation for membranes that extend beneath the center of the foveal avascular zone in patients with AMD. A trial evaluating the laser treatment of subfoveal neovascular membranes in POHS also is contemplated. This chapter describes how to diagnose choroidal neovascular membranes in these two diseases as well as how to treat them with laser photocoagulation.

DIAGNOSIS

Aging Macular Degeneration

A variety of fundus changes occur in AMD, including hard and soft drusen, retinal pigment epithelial atrophy, and retinal pigment epithelial detachments. Ophthalmologists must recognize the symptoms and the clinical and fluorescein angiographic characteristics of each of these changes in order to differentiate them from choroidal neovascularization.[5–7]

Drusen

Drusen appear as round or oval, yellowish deposits beneath the retina. Histopathologic examination reveals PAS-positive deposits lying between the basement membrane of the retinal pigment epithelium (RPE) and Bruch's

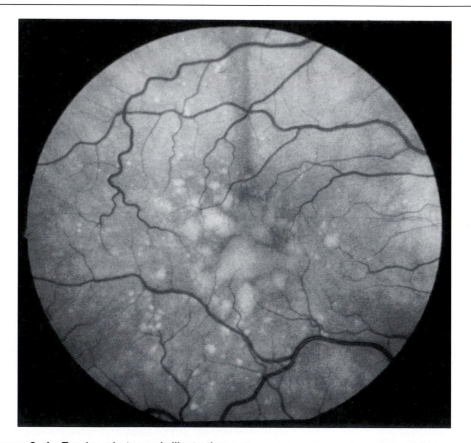

Figure 9–1. Fundus photograph illustrating wet or serous drusen in center of fovea, semisolid drusen parafoveally, and hard drusen around the outskirts, especially inferiorly.

membrane. Sarks has classified drusen into four types: hard drusen, semisolid drusen, soft or serous drusen, and regressing drusen.[8] Hard drusen are small and discrete, with sharp borders. They act as window defects during fluorescein angiography because of overlying thinning of the RPE. Window defects demonstrate early hyperfluorescence and late fading.

Soft or serous drusen are larger, have less discrete or soft edges, and often become confluent. Like RPE detachments, there may be a cruciate pigment pattern over the surface of soft drusen. Fluorescein enters these drusen early and accumulates under the RPE, resembling small serous detachments of the RPE (Fig. 9–1).

Semisolid drusen lie between the two extremes of hard drusen and soft drusen. Regressing drusen appear as the overlying RPE degenerates. These drusen appear whiter and denser on ophthalmoscopy and often are calcified and have irregular margins. Fluorescein dye will accumulate within drusen but will not leak beyond their margins. Late leakage of fluorescein usually indicates a choroidal neovascular membrane.

Often, a choroidal neovascular membrane never develops in patients with drusen. Patients with hard drusen can remain stable or gradually develop retinal pigment epithelial atrophy. Soft drusen, or retinal pigment epithelial detachments, also often collapse into areas of RPE atrophy. These areas may coalesce, resulting in geographic atrophy of the pigment epithelium or dry (atrophic) macular degeneration. These patients usually have a slow progressive visual loss without the abrupt loss of vision and symptoms of metamorphopsia seen in patients with choroidal neovascularization. Although it is uncommon for patients with advanced dry macular degeneration to develop choroidal neovascularization, it is important to evaluate these patients promptly if they develop acute symptoms of visual loss or metamorphopsia.

Retinal Pigment Epithelial Detachments

A retinal pigment epithelial detachment is a separation of the retinal pigment epithelium along with its basement membrane from the underlying Bruch's membrane. Because normally there is strong adherence between the RPE and Bruch's membrane, pigment epithelial detachments usually have sharply defined borders. If fluid separates the pigment epithelium from Bruch's membrane, the detachment is termed "serous." On angiography, there is an early, even filling of the serous detachment, with accumulation of dye causing persistent hyperfluorescence in the late phases (Fig. 9–2). The dye does not leak beyond the confines of the pigment epithelial detachment unless there is an interruption in the continuity of the detached pigment epithelium or, more commonly, choroidal neovascularization. Small pigment epithelial detachments are difficult or impossible to differentiate either clinically or angiographically from large serous drusen.

Patients with serous pigment epithelial detachments usually have mild to moderate losses in visual acuity and may or may not have metamorphopsia, depending on whether there is an overlying neurosensory retinal detachment. Patients over the age of 55 years with retinal pigment epithelial detachments have a high risk of developing choroidal neovascularization.[9–12] Argon photocoagulation, when applied over the surface of the detached epithelium, may cause the detachment to flatten. The only controlled prospective study, however, of eyes with serous RPE detachments found that argon-treated eyes suffered an early deterioration in visual acuity more often than did untreated eyes.[9] The differences were significant at the 3-, 6-, and 9-month follow-up visits. Later, the untreated eyes also deteriorated but never became worse than the treated eyes. There was also no difference in the incidence of subsequent choroidal neovascularization between treated and untreated eyes. This study has been criticized because it contained some eyes that already had choroidal

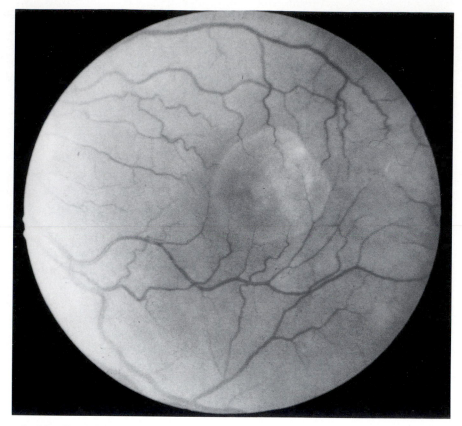

Figure 9–2A. Fundus photograph illustrating serous retinal pigment epithelial detachment with typical sharp borders and no sign of neovascularization.

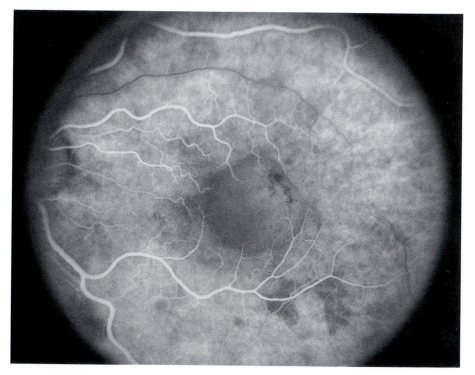

Figure 9–2B. Early homogeneous filling of the RPE detachment.

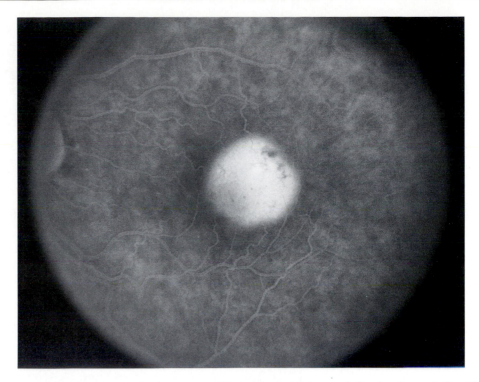

Figure 9–2C. Late hyperfluorescence with no leakage beyond the borders of the RPE detachment.

neovascularization at the time of treatment and because heavy confluent argon blue-green photocoagulation was placed over large areas of the detachments. Thus, the best treatment for serous detachments of the RPE is not known.

When there is underlying choroidal neovascularization, pigment epithelial detachments typically do not fill uniformly. Hyperfluorescence, or hot spots, during fluorescein angiography caused by leakage from neovascularization may be noted beneath the turbid fluid of the detachment. Often, neovascularization is present in a notch that interrupts the smooth round border of the RPE detachment (Fig. 9–3). Hemorrhage from neovascularization beneath the surface of the pigment epithelium can cause an area of hypofluorescence during angiography. Extensive hemorrhage appears as a slate gray, dome-shaped lesion called a "hemorrhagic pigment epithelial detachment." Usually, some of the hemorrhage will dissect from beneath the pigment epithelium under the neurosensory retina and appear as a bright red subretinal hemorrhage. Because it is difficult to define the full extent of the choroidal neovascular membrane beneath hemorrhage or turbid fluid, it is difficult to treat these patients. The prognosis is poor with or without treatment, and it remains unknown whether photocoagulation reduces visual loss.

Choroidal Neovascularization

The diagnosis of choroidal neovascularization in patients with AMD is important because it is the main cause of visual loss and because studies have shown that laser photocoagulation reduces the rate of this loss.[1,4] Patients with dry or atrophic macular degeneration suffer a gradual, long-term visual loss without metamorphopsia, which may not be amenable to treatment. A

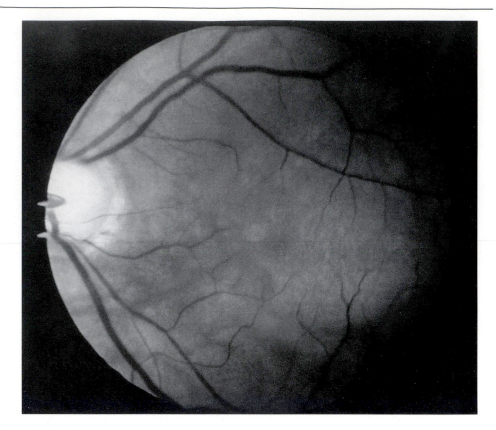

Figure 9–3A. Fundus photograph illustrating RPE detachment with notched border on the inferonasal edge secondary to a choroidal neovascular membrane.

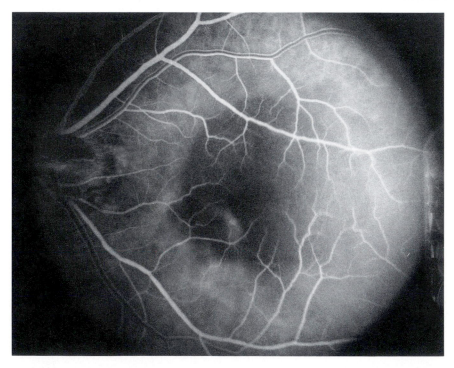

Figure 9–3B. Early hypofluorescence in notch from subretinal neovascular membrane.

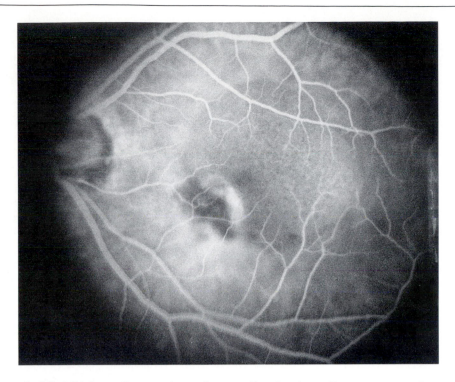

Figure 9–3C. Midphase fluorescein angiogram showing hyperfluorescent membrane and early pooling in pigment epithelial detachment.

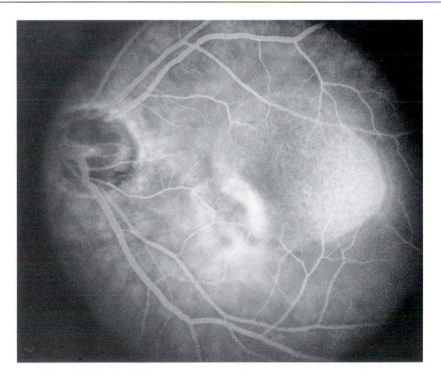

Figure 9–3D. Late leakage from notch and filled RPE detachment.

patient with a choroidal neovascular membrane will typically note a more abrupt visual loss, metamorphopsia, and sometimes a paracentral scotoma. Metamorphopsia is a bending or distortion of vision that usually is noticed when viewing straight objects, such as door edges or telephone poles. The patient should be questioned carefully concerning symptoms of metamorphopsia because it usually indicates a neurosensory retinal detachment secondary to the presence of neovascularization. The Amsler grid examination is helpful in outlining the extent of the scotoma and distortion.

Patients with macular degeneration are examined initially with the indirect ophthalmoscope, mainly to rule out other causes of visual loss. The posterior pole can then be scanned with the direct ophthalmoscope or with the 78 D or 90 D lens at the slit lamp. These will allow the clinician to get an overall view of the posterior pole and alert the ophthalmologist to areas that deserve closer study. In order to detect a subtle serous detachment or choroidal neovascularization, the macula must be examined under high magnification with good stereopsis. A Hruby lens is effective, but the best method of examination is with the planoconcave (pancake) contact lens or the similar Yannuzzi lens. This lens should be used after fundus photography because the necessary topical anesthetic and gonioscopic coupling solution will decrease corneal clarity. The planoconcave contact lens is superior to the central aperture of the Goldmann three-mirror lens for examining the posterior pole.

A choroidal neovascular membrane (CNVM) is typically darker or grayish in color compared to the surrounding drusen or areas of retinal pigment epithelial atrophy. The membrane lies deep to the retina, and there is often a pigmented or depigmented border along its edges. Sometimes the only sign of a CNVM is a localized fuzziness caused by the overlying neurosensory retinal detachment (Fig. 9–4). In this localized area, the deeper retinal and pig-

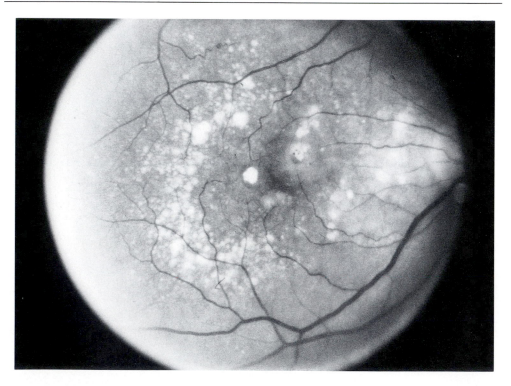

Figure 9–4A. Fundus photograph showing subtle choroidal neovascularization. Note grayish fuzziness and pinpoint hemorrhages superior nasal to fovea.

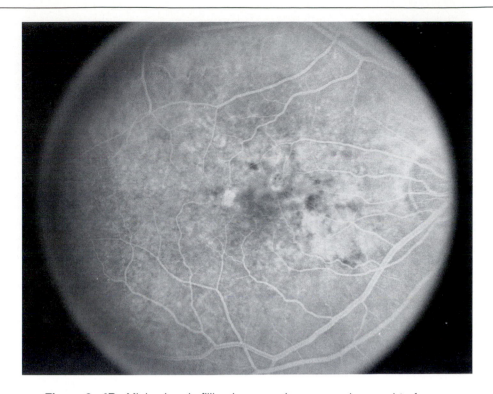

Figure 9–4B. Minimal early filling in a round area superior nasal to fovea.

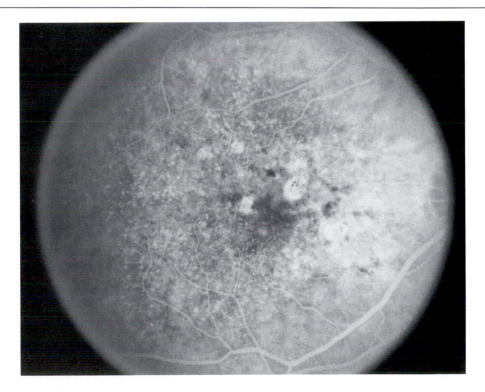

Figure 9–4C. Midphase angiogram showing complete filling and early leakage.

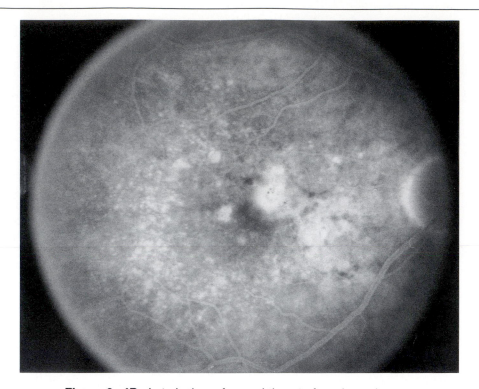

Figure 9–4D. Late leakage from subtle extrafoveal membrane.

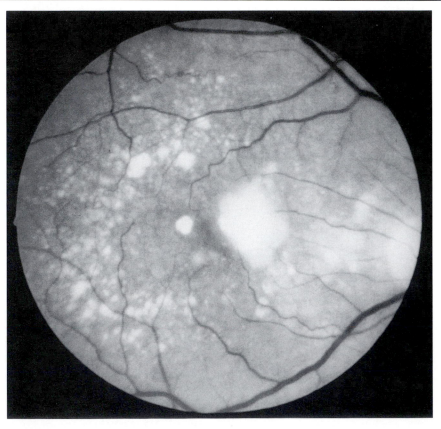

Figure 9–4E. Photograph immediately after heavy argon green photocoagulation to neovascular membrane.

ment epithelial structures are obscured in contrast to the other areas of the macula, where drusen and pigment epithelial atrophy can be seen and defined clearly. The presence of subpigment epithelial or subretinal hemorrhage is almost a sure sign of neovascularization. There is often only a small fleck of hemorrhage present, however, so the fundus must be examined carefully and with a high degree of clinical suspicion. The presence of subretinal exudate also indicates choroidal neovascularization but is uncommon. The presence of a neurosensory retinal detachment, which is best seen using contact lens biomicroscopy, typically indicates choroidal neovascularization.

A CNVM usually can be detected by clinical examination alone. Fluorescein angiography is not required in patients who obviously have only drusen or dry macular degeneration and no new symptoms. An angiogram should be performed if there are any areas suspicious for a CNVM or if the patient describes new symptoms. Fluorescein angiograms often are difficult to interpret in the elderly patient because of extensive drusen and pigmentary abnormalities and because of haziness due to media opacities. A high-quality stereoscopic angiogram is important to detect the presence of a neovascular membrane and the location of the fovea.

Choroidal neovascular membranes typically have a round or oval shape. They are fed from the choroidal vasculature and, therefore, fill early in the angiogram. Well-visualized membranes often have a lacy or cartwheel appearance. The membranes continue to fill in the midphases of the angiogram and leak late. A thin rim of hypofluorescence often surrounds the membrane.

Sometimes, neovascular membranes are difficult to visualize because they fill and leak slowly or are surrounded by background hyperfluorescence from drusen or retinal pigment epithelial atrophy. A technique for reading fluorescein angiograms is to first cut the negatives into strips of six pictures each and to include stereo pairs on the same strip. Positives of the photographs also may be used, but negatives have better resolution. On examining the negatives, the examiner should remember that the fluorescein dye is black rather than white. The strips are put into plastic holders and then onto a light box. Stereo pairs are examined through a $4\times$ aerial viewer (Air Photo Supply, Yonkers, NY) or high plus (aphakic) glasses. In eyes in which a CNVM is difficult to visualize, it is helpful to study first a late pair of frames to locate areas suspicious for leakage. Then backtrack by jumping one or several rows of photographs into the midphase and early phase of the angiogram. Try to fit the area of leakage into a round or oval area seen in the early phases that corresponds to the CNVM. Often, a hypofluorescent rim helps to define the membrane.

Sometimes there is not a clearly definable structure that fills with fluorescein, then leaks. Instead, there is mottling of the RPE along with a few hot spots that slowly leak fluorescein dye late in the angiogram. These findings have been termed "oozes" and probably represent occult neovascular membranes that are filling very slowly or whose leakage is being restricted by the overlying RPE. Helpful clues in detecting the entire area of the neovascular membrane include the hypofluorescent border or an area of elevated RPE seen on the stereo pairs. A careful examination with a contact lens usually will reveal a nodular structure deep to the retina that can be differentiated clearly from the surrounding normal tissue and corresponds to the area of leakage or RPE elevation on the angiogram.

Findings in the Presumed Ocular Histoplasmosis Syndrome

Findings in POHS include peripapillary scarring, peripheral discrete (punched-out) scars, and the development of choroidal neovascularization within the macula. Spores of *Histoplasma capsulatum* are inhaled and first cause a localized pulmonary infection. The organism is then disseminated into the bloodstream, causing lesions in the viscera and choroiditis, with subsequent scarring in the eye. Later, most often in early to midadulthood, choroidal neovascularization occurs in the macula, usually contiguous with an old histoplasmosis scar. The cause of this later neovascularization is unknown.

Histoplasmosis patients with choroidal neovascularization develop typical symptoms of decreased vision, scotomas, and metamorphopsia. Unlike AMD, the surrounding retina in histoplasmosis patients is normal, allowing subretinal membranes to be visualized more easily. Choroidal neovascular membranes in POHS usually are small or moderately sized, round or oval in shape, and often surrounded by a band of pigmentation. There is an overlying serous neurosensory retinal detachment and, typically, subretinal hemorrhage.

Patient Selection

The Macular Photocoagulation Studies have shown that argon and krypton laser treatment reduces the risk of visual loss in patients with extrafoveal or juxtafoveal neovascular membranes in patients with either AMD or POHS. Therefore, it is very important not to miss CNVMs in these patients. Careful stereoscopic examinations of the fundus under high magnification, as well as fluorescein angiography, is indicated in any patient with new findings or symptoms.

Currently, there is no definitive proof that laser photocoagulation is efficacious in patients with neovascular membranes that extend beneath the center of the foveal avascular zone in AMD or POHS. Bressler et al.[13] found that nearly all patients with large subfoveal membranes attributable to AMD deteriorate to 20/200 or worse, including 75% of patients who initially had an acuity of 20/100 or better.[14] The natural history of subfoveal membranes in POHS also appears to be poor. Therefore, treatment may be justified in these foveal patients if it results in a small, dry, stable central scar and allows the patient to better use low vision aids. On the other hand, foveal treatment will result in the destruction of all foveal cones in that area, including those cones that may still be functional. The most current arm of the MPS dealing with this subset of patients has terminated recruitment of patients with AMD and subfoveal membranes. These patients were randomized so that half received either argon green or krypton red laser treatment, and the other half received no treatment. The results of this study have yet to be announced. The MPS Group also is contemplating randomizing patients with POHS and subfoveal membranes to a similar protocol of laser treatment vs observation.

LASER TREATMENT

If the laser treatment does not cover the entire extent of the CNVM, it usually will recur after treatment. Therefore, it is most important to define carefully the entire extent of the neovascularization. First, study negatives (although positives also can be used) of the fluorescein angiogram on a light box through 4× aerial viewers or aphakic glasses. Stereoscopic angiograms are necessary to visualize subtle areas of RPE elevation. In AMD patients, hyperfluorescent spots or RPE elevation contiguous with more obvious areas of neovascular membrane usually indicates extension of the neovascularization and should be treated.[15] On the other hand, areas of RPE under a serous detachment surrounding a membrane also can hyperfluoresce a bit late in the angiogram and do not necessarily mean extension of the neovascularization. Often, there is a pigment ring or hypofluorescent border surrounding the membrane, which can help to define its border. Choroidal neovascular membranes in histoplasmosis usually are more easy to define because they fill and leak briskly, are usually bordered by pigment, and have normal surrounding RPE to contrast with the adjacent membrane.

The following treatment technique is that used by the MPS Group.[1-4] It is the only treatment method that has been proven effective and is now used by most retinal experts. The goal of this treatment is to cover the area of neovascularization with intense argon green or krypton red laser photocoagulation (Table 9–1). The end points are a chalky pure white burn with the argon laser and a slightly less off-white burn with the krypton red laser. If the CNVM is more than 200 μm from the center of the fovea, the laser treatment should overlap the edges of the membrane by 100 μm. If the CNVM is closer than 200 μm, the treatment should still cover and overlap the CNVM, but just barely, in order to spare functioning foveal cones.

Clinicians previously began treatment by outlining the neovascular membrane with small (50 or 100 μm) spots of argon laser. They found, however, that it was difficult to achieve intense uniform coverage of the membrane using these small spots. In addition, the smaller spots increased the risk of rupture of Bruch's membrane and hemorrhage, especially when using the krypton red laser. Therefore, a spreading technique of treatment was developed that uses larger (200 μm or more) and longer (0.2 sec or more) laser burns.[16,17] The laser beam is aimed just inside the border of the membrane and is activated. The burn enlarges and spreads over the edge of the CNVM. This spreading technique results in a more uniform and intense treatment than the technique that first outlined the membrane with very small spots. The spreading technique is now preferred and is described here.

A frame of the angiogram that has good resolution and shows complete filling of, but not yet leakage from, the CNVM is magnified on a viewer next to the patient. Usually, this is a photograph from the early or mid (about 25 sec) phase of the angiogram. The patient is then examined at the slit lamp

---

TABLE 9–1. Laser Photocoagulation for Choroidal Neovascular Membranes

Spot Size	200–500 μm
Duration of Burn	0.2–0.5 sec
Initial Power Setting	200 mW
Wavelength	Argon green (514 nm)
	Krypton red[a] (647 nm)
Contact Lens	Planoconcave (pancake) or Yannuzzi
Anesthesia	Retrobulbar (usually) or topical

Goal: White, intense laser burns should be confluent and cover the entire extent of the choroidal neovascular membrane. Laser burns should overlap edges of the neovascular complex by 100 μm unless closer than 200 μm from the center of the foveal avascular zone, when the edges should be just covered. Use the spreading technique to allow intense and uniform treatment and increase the power setting in 50 mW increments until the desired intensity is achieved.

[a]Krypton red may be used in place of argon green when the neovascular complex is not easily visualized secondary to overlying subretinal or intraretinal hemorrhage or located within the foveal avascular zone.

using a contact lens. The clinical examination is repeatedly compared with the magnified angiogram frame, and the area of needed treatment is planned carefully. In difficult cases, this comparison may require as much as 10 to 15 minutes of intense concentration. A drawing from the angiogram showing the area of neovascularization and important landmarks often is helpful. The patient is counseled concerning the risks vs benefits of treatment and the results of the MPS. The patient should be told of the resulting scotoma from laser photocoagulation and that the recurrence rate (especially in AMD) is high. Thus, even in adequately treated neovascular membranes, the long-term prognosis is guarded.

Usually, a retrobulbar anesthetic is given to obtain adequate anesthesia and akinesia. It may be unnecessary in a cooperative patient who has good vision in the opposite eye, which can be used for fixation during the treatment. The Yannuzzi lens is a modified planoconcave (pancake) lens with a larger surrounding flange. This flange allows the clinician to push on the globe with the lens in order to hold it steady and to elevate the intraocular pressure. These features make the Yannuzzi a preferred lens for treatment of choroidal neovascularization. The patient is seated comfortably at the slit lamp and asked to fixate if possible with the opposite eye. The patient should be assured that although many spots may be used to treat the CNVM, the spots are small and frequently are used to retreat the same area repeatedly to ensure adequate treatment. Therefore, the final area of treatment will remain small.

In the MPS, argon blue-green laser was used for treatment of extrafoveal membranes (greater than or equal to 200 μm) and krypton red laser for treatment of membranes closer than 200 μm to the center of the foveal avascular zone. The blue component of the argon blue-green laser should now be filtered out because of its preferential absorption by macular xanthophyll. Both the argon green and krypton red lasers can effectively destroy choroidal neovascularization. The krypton red laser seems to be gaining popularity because it appears to result in deeper burns with less overlying inner retinal damage. The spread of the krypton laser may be easier to control, and the membrane and other landmarks are easier to visualize during treatment because of less inner retinal opacification. Krypton red definitely should be used if there is surrounding or overlying hemorrhage, based on its absorption characteristics that allow less absorption by hemoglobin.[18–20] Argon green probably should be used for the treatment of red or white membranes because krypton red requires pigmentation for adequate absorption.

The argon green or krypton red laser settings are 200 μm, 0.2 sec or longer, and 150 mW. An edge of the membrane away from the fovea is treated first, and the power is increased until a white burn is obtained. At this time, there are two techniques to treat the foveal edge. Many clinicians use the first technique, which is to begin with less intense spots and repeatedly retreat over these spots to achieve the desired final intense burn. The advantage of this technique is that there is less chance of an overly intense burn with perforation of Bruch's membrane or hemorrhage. The clinician can slowly increase the area and whiteness of the burn. The disadvantage is that the clinician is treating repeatedly close to the fovea, which increases the risk of spread of the burns or even an errant spot. Another disadvantage is that once the tissue turns slightly white, further absorption of the laser may be very difficult.

The second technique is used more often at The University of Iowa. The location of the neovascular process is documented carefully using biomicroscopy (Fig. 9–5A). The power of the laser is increased until a white burn is achieved that is close to but slightly less than the desired end point (Fig. 9–5B). The foveal edge is then treated with this fairly intense burn (Fig. 9–5C). The advantage of this technique is that the clinician can visualize the mem-

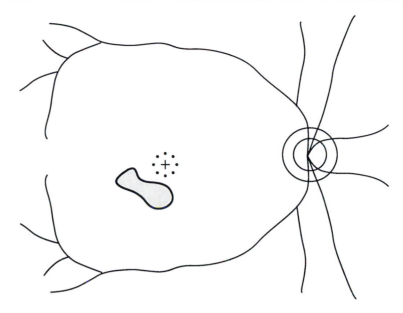

Figure 9–5A. Macular region. Area in box contains extrafoveal neovascular membrane, which is enlarged in the following figures.

brane and then go after it with an intense burn. Fewer burns are required, lessening the spread of the treatment or the risk of an errant shot. The disadvantage is that areas of the retina and membrane can absorb laser variably, and some of these burns will be too intense and cause a rupture of Bruch's membrane or a hemorrhage. A safety factor is to use an energy that causes a burn slightly less than the desired end point. In this way, if an area of retina absorbs more energy, the burn will reach the desired end point but will not

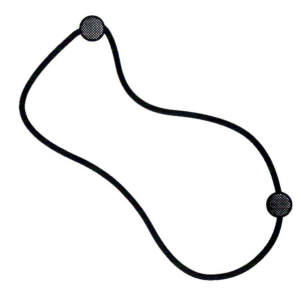

Figure 9–5B. Extrafoveal neovascular membrane with test burns on superior or inferior edges that are increased until a white burn that is slightly less than the desired end point is achieved.

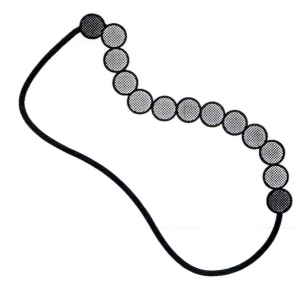

Figure 9–5C. Spreading of treatment burns over the foveal edge of the neovascular membrane. This neovascular membrane is over 200 μm from the fovea, and, therefore, the center of the burn is placed directly on the edge of the membrane.

be excessive. On the other hand, it is simple to go over the lighter burns once or twice with this slightly lower setting to achieve the final desired degree of whiteness.

Some techniques include outlining the entire border of the membrane first and then filling in this border. If this technique is employed, it is better to complete the foveal edge of the treatment first. First, treat the very edge, and then immediately retreat this edge until the desired whiteness is achieved. Put a few more rows of burns inside the treatment along the foveal edge, check this edge for adequacy, and then be done with it (Fig. 9–5D). It is unwise to treat inadequately along one border, then move to other borders, and then go back to the original area. This jumping type of treatment necessitates the identification of landmarks over and over again rather than just once. The clinician will end up placing the most critical treatment along the foveal edge at the end of the treatment when the patient (and physician) is fatigued and the landmarks are obscured by corneal haze and previous treatment.

A better technique is to try to identify initially the margins of the neovascular membrane and then be aggressive by overlapping this membrane with treatment (Fig. 9–5C, D) to ensure adequate coverage of the membrane. The surgeon who is too timid initially may end up not being certain of having covered the membrane and may either discontinue treatment and not achieve adequate treatment along the foveal edge or go over and over the edge of the previous treatment until it spreads further into the fovea than was intended or necessary. The foveal edge should be overlapped by 100 μm if it is more than 200 μm from the fovea. If the membrane is closer than 200 μm from the fovea, just cover its edge—but again try to be certain that complete treatment is accomplished.

Once you have treated the foveal side of the membrane, you may treat the nonfoveal borders. Overlap the nonfoveal borders by 100 μm and finally fill in the center within the outline of spots (Fig. 9–5E). Increase the spot size, duration, and intensity of burns and go over the same area until a uniform chalky white (argon) or white (krypton) lesion is attained (Figs. 9–5E, 9–6, and

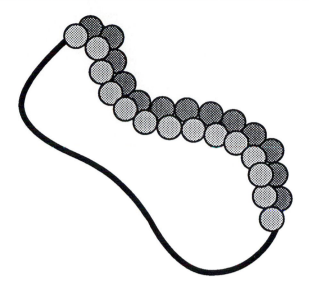

Figure 9–5D. A second row of treatment burns is added over and inside the original row of burns.

9–7). It is important to achieve an intense burn even if you must retreat the center five or more times. These large, long duration burns are very safe.

Finally, recheck all of the borders of the treatment by carefully comparing them to the magnified frame of the fluorescein angiogram. This is very tedious at the end of treatment, but it often picks up areas of inadequate coverage or intensity, which can then be retreated immediately. Occasionally, you will be unsure whether you have covered the foveal edge and would like just a little

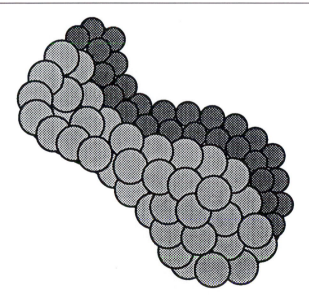

Figure 9–5E. The entire neovascular membrane has been treated using 200 to 500 μm long duration burns. It should be as uniformly white as possible.

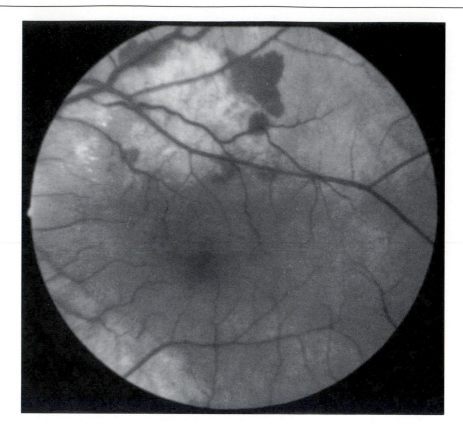

Figure 9–6A. Fundus photograph showing extrafoveal choroidal neovascular membrane superior to fovea.

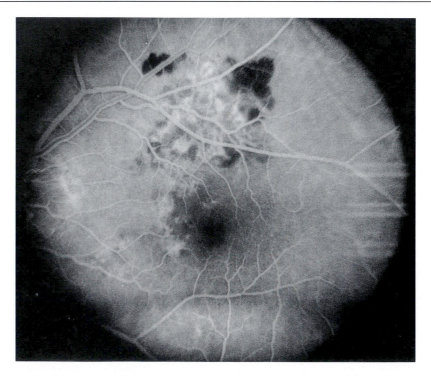

Figure 9–6B. Fluorescein angiogram showing filling of membrane and blockage by blood.

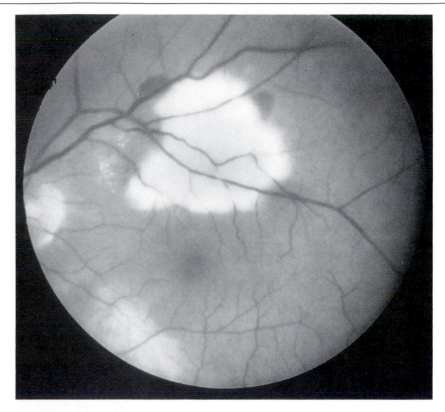

Figure 9–6C. Immediate posttreatment photograph after argon photocoagulation.

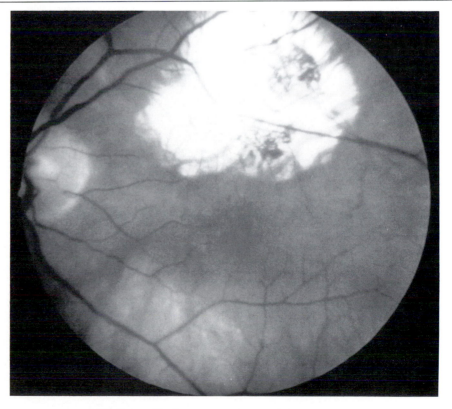

Figure 9–6D. Chorioretinal scar after treatment.

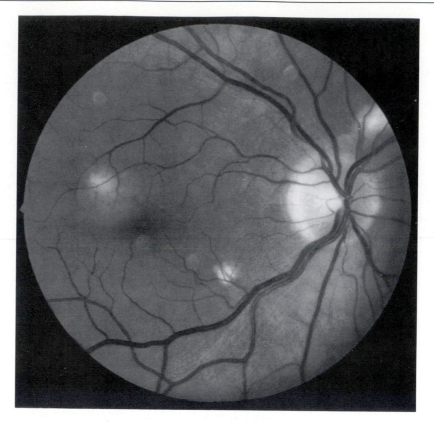

Figure 9–7A. Fundus photograph of POHS patient with choroidal neovascular membrane superior temporal to fovea.

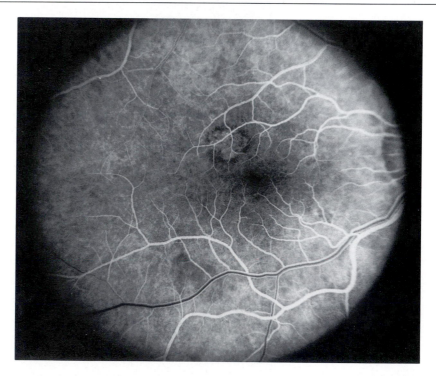

Figure 9–7B. Fluorescein angiogram showing extrafoveal neovascular membrane.

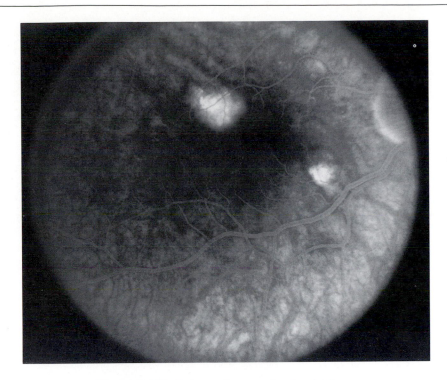

Figure 9–7C. Late angiogram showing leakage.

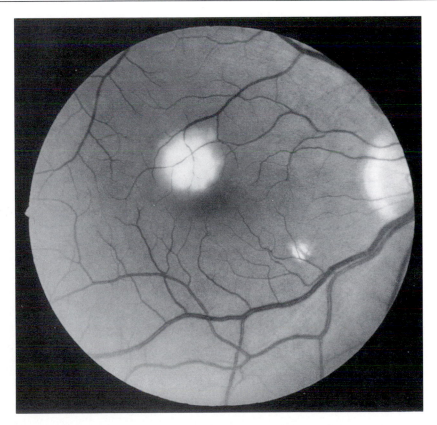

Figure 9–7D. Photograph taken immediately after argon green laser photocoagulation.

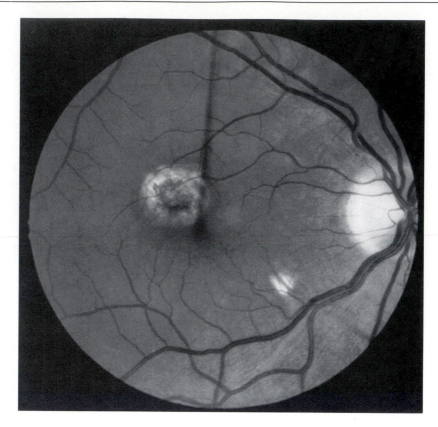

Figure 9–7E. Chorioretinal scar 3 months after treatment. Amsler grid defect is stable, and visual acuity is 20/25.

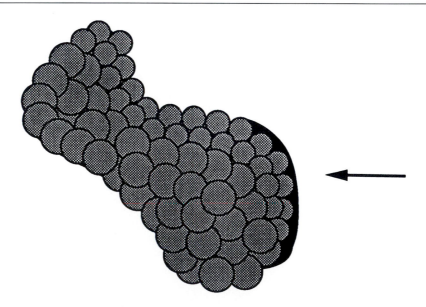

Figure 9–8A. In this example, the inferior foveal edge of the membrane has not been treated adequately (*arrow*).

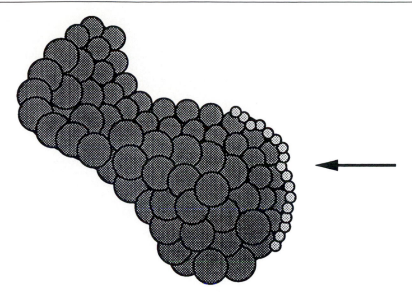

Figure 9–8B. Additional coverage has been added using 50 to 100 μm spot sizes along the edge of the prior treatment zone.

bit more treatment there (Fig. 9–8A). Usually, additional burns will not cause whitening of the RPE until the laser is aimed outside of the previous treatment. If a 200 μm spot size is used, this will result in at least 200 μm or more of treatment along the foveal edge, which will be excessive unless you grossly undertreated the membrane initially. Therefore, it is recommended to turn the laser to a 50 or 100 μm spot size and decrease the power. Usually, you can then carefully dance along the foveal edge of the prior treatment area, gradually increasing the power until you obtain the additional desired coverage (Fig. 9–8B). It is better to be aggressive initially and cover the membrane than to perform these laser gymnastics late in the treatment session.

Posttreatment color and red-free photographs should be taken if desired. The eye is then patched if a retrobulbar anesthetic was used. The patient is advised that a new scotoma will be created from this laser treatment and that vision may be more blurred than before. This blurring and scotoma should stabilize by the second day after treatment and then remain the same or gradually improve. The patient should be told repeatedly to return promptly if there is any worsening of visual acuity or new metamorphopsias seen on frequent Amsler grid testing. Patients return in 2 to 3 weeks for an examination and a posttreatment angiogram. A posttreatment angiogram must be examined meticulously to determine whether there is persistence of the neovascular membrane. A persistent or recurrent neovascular membrane should be treated promptly if it does not extend beneath the center of the fovea. Patients are usually evaluated in another month and in another 2 to 3 months thereafter. After that, they usually can be seen every 6 to 12 months or discharged to their referring physicians. At every visit, the patient should be given an Amsler grid and instructed to return promptly if there are any new symptoms of metamorphopsia.

SUMMARY

Patients with aging macular degeneration or presumed ocular histoplasmosis and choroidal neovascular membranes not beneath the center of the fovea should be treated with either heavy argon green or krypton red photocoagulation. It is most important to define carefully the extent of the neovascularization before treatment and then to cover it with intense laser burns. The efficacy of laser photocoagulation for AMD or POHS patients whose membranes extend beneath the center of the fovea is still unknown and awaits the results of the Macular Photocoagulation Studies.

REFERENCES

1. Macular Photocoagulation Study Group: Argon laser photocoagulation for senile macular degeneration: results of a randomized clinical trial. *Arch Ophthalmol* 1982; 100:912–918.
2. Macular Photocoagulation Study Group: Argon laser photocoagulation for ocular histoplasmosis: results of a randomized clinical trial. *Arch Ophthalmol* 1983; 101:1347–1357.
3. Macular Photocoagulation Study Group: Krypton laser photocoagulation for neovascular lesions of ocular histoplasmosis: results of a randomized clinical trial. *Arch Ophthalmol* 1987;105:1499–1507.
4. Macular Photocoagulation Study Group: Krypton laser photocoagulation for neovascular lesions of age-related macular degeneration: results of a randomized clinical trial. *Arch Ophthalmol* 1990;108:816–824.
5. Gass JDM: Choroidal diseases causing localized (disciform) detachment of the retina and pigment epithelium. In: *Stereoscopic Atlas of Macular Disease*. St. Louis, MO: CV Mosby Co; 1977.
6. Gass JDM: Drusen and disciform macular degeneration. *Trans Am Ophthalmol Soc* 1972;70:409–436.
7. Gragoudas ES, Chandra SR, Freidman E, Klein ML, Van Buskirk M: Disciform degeneration of the macula. *Arch Ophthalmol* 1976;94:755–757.
8. Sarks SH: Drusen and their relationship to senile macular degeneration. *Aust J Ophthalmol* 1980;8:117–130.
9. The Moorfields Macular Study Group: Retinal pigment epithelial detachments in the elderly: a controlled trial of argon laser photocoagulation. *Br J Ophthalmol* 1982; 66:1–16.
10. Klein ML, Obertynski H, Patz A, Fine SL, Kini M: Follow-up study of detachment of the retinal pigment epithelium. *Br J Ophthalmol* 1980;64:412–416.
11. Meredith TA, Braley RE, Aaberg TM: Natural history of serous detachments of the retinal pigment epithelium. *Am J Ophthalmol* 1979;88:643–651.
12. Lewis ML: Idiopathic serous detachment of the retinal pigment epithelium. *Arch Ophthalmol* 1978;96:620–624.
13. Bressler SB, Bressler NM, Fine SL, Hillis A, Murphy RP, Olk RJ, Patz A: Natural course of choroidal neovascular membranes within the foveal avascular zone in senile macular degeneration. *Am J Ophthalmol* 1982;93:157–163.
14. Kleiner RC, Ratner CM, Enger C, Fine SL: Subfoveal neovascularization in the ocular histoplasmosis syndrome. *Retina* 1988;8:225–229.
15. Bressler NM, Frost LA, Bressler SB, et al: Natural course of poorly defined choroidal neovascularization associated with macular degeneration. *Arch Ophthalmol* 1988; 106:1537–1542.
16. Singerman LJ: Red krypton laser therapy of macular and retinal vascular diseases. *Retina* 1982;2:15–18.
17. Yannuzzi LA: Krypton red laser photocoagulation for subretinal neovascularization. *Retina* 1982;2:29–46.
18. Marshall J, Bird AC: A comparative histopathological study of argon and krypton laser indications of the retina. *Br J Ophthalmol* 1979;63:657–668.
19. Trempe CL, Mainster MA, Pomerantzeff O, Avila MP, Jalkh AE, Wieter JJ, McMeel JW, Schepens CL: Macular photocoagulation: optimal wavelength selection. *Ophthalmology* 1982;89:721–728.
20. Yannuzzi LA, Shakin JL: Krypton red laser photocoagulation of the ocular fundus. *Retina* 1982;2:1–14.

CHAPTER 10

Selected Vascular Disorders of the Fundus

Stephen R. Russell and Vernon M. Hermsen

ANGIOMATOSIS RETINAE

INTRODUCTION

The term "angiomatosis retinae" was first applied by von Hippel to red-orange intraretinal capillary hemangiomas typically perfused by a prominent dilated retinal artery and drained by a dilated, sometimes tortuous retinal vein.[1] After Lindau's classic article in 1927, which emphasized the association of these retinal angiomas with tumors of the central nervous system and visceral organs,[2] investigators have described a plethora of accompanying lesions of von Hippel-Lindau disease (VHL). These include cerebellar and spinal hemangioblastomas, pheochromocytomas, and clear cell renal carcinomas.[3] The proportion of patients who have retinal angiomas and who are confirmed to have VHL has increased to greater than 50%. This is due, in part, to the use of more sensitive noninvasive imaging techniques, such as CT scanning, MR scanning, and diagnostic ultrasonography. Von Hippel-Lindau disease, an autosomal dominant disorder, has been linked to a locus on chromosome 3p25, near the human homologue of the RAF 1 oncogene.[4,5] The spontaneous mutation rate at this locus is probably very low, although isolated retinal angiomas may exist.[6]

The potentially lethal manifestations of von Hippel-Lindau disease dictate regular lifelong ophthalmoscopic, neurologic, and endocrinologic surveillance in all patients and their family members at risk (Table 10–1). Silent tumors and cysts may require several decades to become evident. Therefore, the diagnosis of VHL in all patients with retinal angiomas remains uncertain unless excluded by a thorough autopsy[3] and family evaluation. Retinal angiomas have been documented in a 1-day-old neonate[7] and in sexagenarians thought to have normal fundi.[8] Therefore, patients should be advised to consult with an internist, neurologist, and medical geneticist on diagnosis of a retinal angioma.

DIAGNOSIS

Meticulous indirect ophthalmoscopy should include scleral depression of the entire peripheral retina. Questionable lesions may be further examined using a Goldmann three-mirror contact lens. Fluorescein angiography is rarely useful for screening but is quite helpful in evaluating suspicious lesions.

TABLE 10–1. SUGGESTED SCREENING PROTOCOL FOR PATIENTS WITH RETINAL ANGIOMAS[a]

Indirect ophthalmoscopy with scleral depression annually for those at risk and at least once every 6 months for affected members

Annual examination by medical internist or pediatrician
   Full physical, with particular attention to blood pressure, lying and standing
   24-hour urine collection for urinary catecholamines and metanephrines
   Plasma catecholamines if blood pressure is elevated or postural hypotension is present.
   Abdominal CT scan if biochemical abnormalities are found

Annual neurologic examination with particular attention to any cerebellar signs
   Baseline CT scan in late teens or early twenties
   CT scan repeated if any suspicious neurologic findings

Annual ultrasound of kidneys, pancreas, and liver
   CT scan or IV pyelogram of kidneys, if indicated

Medical genetics consultation on diagnosis

[a]After Ridley M, Green J, Johnson G: *Can J Ophthalmol* 1986;21:276–283.

Retinal angiomas are usually endophytic, extending from the retinal substance, and occur as homogeneous or variegated red-orange or white elevated nodules, or both. Each may have a dilated feeding artery and a large draining vein (Fig. 10–1). Retinal edema or exudate may surround the tumor or accumulate in the macula as an exaggerated exudative response or Coats'-like reaction. Incipient lesions, which are ophthalmoscopically visible as capillary dilations, resemble diabetic microaneurysms.[8] In addition, prominent dilated capillary shunting, similar to intraretinal microangiopathy (IRMA), may be seen. In most cases, angiomas enlarge slowly, which, in turn, may compromise the eye and complicate treatment. Visual acuity may be affected by retinal edema, serous retinal detachment with exudation, or traction[9] or combined traction and rhegmatogenous retinal detachment[10] involving the angioma. Secondary neovascular glaucoma may complicate prolonged detachment. Because retinal lesions progress, they should be treated as soon as feasible.

In contrast to retinal lesions, peripapillary angiomas are usually exophytic and appear as ruddy elevations of the optic nerve margins. They also may be associated with surrounding retinal edema and exudate. Dilated feeding arteries and tortuous draining veins are uncommon. Peripapillary angiomas may be confused with subretinal neovascular membranes, papilledema, osteoma, or combined retinal pigment epithelial-vascular hamartomas.[11] Photocoagulation of peripapillary angiomas is problematic, since optic disc damage may result. Peripapillary angiomas typically enlarge over months to years. When exudate or serous detachment affects visual function, treatment may be considered.

Fluorescein angiography is the most useful diagnostic test for evaluating suspicious lesions. Both retinal and peripapillary angiomas demonstrate filling of the retinal capillaries in the arterial phase and leak fluorescein profusely.

LASER TREATMENT

Treatment Alternatives

Retinal angiomas less than 1 DD in size that are accessible to photocoagulation generally respond well.[3] Intermediate sized angiomas (1–2.5 DD) may be treated with photocoagulation or cryopexy.[3,13] External cryopexy is preferred when the angioma is too anterior to photocoagulate, too thick to allow complete photocoagulative ablation, or associated with extensive serous retinal detachment (usually >2 DD) precluding adequate energy absorption (due to separation from melanin in the retinal pigment epithelium). Angiomas larger than 2.5 DD may respond poorly to either photocoagulation or cryopexy. In these cases, retinal artery ligation,[12] eye wall resection,[14] or transscleral penetrating diathermy[15] may be considered. Larger angiomas may develop associated fibrocellular proliferation, which may necessitate consultation with a vitreoretinal surgeon.

Wavelength Selection

Numerous reports have documented the response of angiomas to argon laser photocoagulation.[3,6,9,11,12] Treatment typically has been directed to the angioma surface and not to the feeder vessels. However, Nicholson has successfully applied argon photocoagulation to occlude afferent retinal arteries following elevation of the intraocular pressure above ocular arterial perfusion pressure by forcing the therapeutic contact lens against the cornea.[16] Because of its relatively high hemoglobin absorption, dye yellow (577 nm) has a theoretical advantage in ablating these vascular lesions.[17] Photocoagulation with

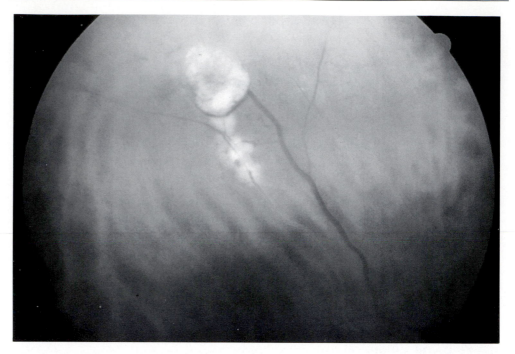

A

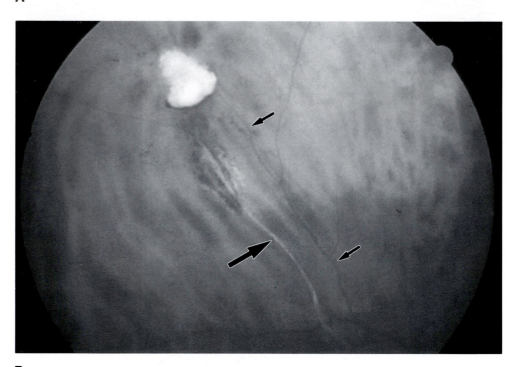

B

Figure 10–1. Serial fundus photographs of dye yellow photocoagulation of a retinal angioma on a feeding artery. Note the vascularity within the tumor and the prominent feeding artery and draining vein. **A.** One hundred eighty-one burns were applied to the artery (240 mW, 0.2 sec, 200 μm). **B.** Two months later, the feeding artery has developed a sclerotic wall that extends to its proximal branch point (*large arrow*), the caliber of the draining vein is dramatically reduced (*small arrows*), and no perfusion is seen within the angioma. Repeat fundus fluorescein angiography failed to demonstrate any significant vascular leakage. *(Photographs courtesy of Christopher F. Blodi, M.D., The University of Iowa.)*

dye yellow (577 nm) light has been shown to be more effective in occluding afferent arteries and is at least as effective as argon photocoagulation for surface ablation.[18]

Treatment Techniques

Angiomas 1 DD and smaller may be treated following topical anesthesia (Table 10–2). Larger lesions usually will require retrobulbar anesthesia because of the moderately intense power required. One drop of topical anesthesia is instilled into the fornix, and a Rodenstock or three-mirror contact lens is applied. When using argon green (514 nm), treatment should be directed to the tumor surface. Confluent photocoagulation is applied to the angioma surface to obtain a white lesion. Dye yellow photocoagulation may be directed to the angioma surface, the feeding artery, or both structures. The treatment goal is to obtain a blanched tumor in the case of arteriolar treatment or moderately white photocoagulation of the tumor surface itself or both. Treating the retina immediately adjacent to the angioma may be of benefit in some cases to prevent the formation of collateral arterial perfusion. Photocoagulation of the draining retinal vein should be avoided.

Follow-up and Complications

Patients should be followed at intervals of 3 to 6 weeks until complete ablation of angiomas is observed. Complications that follow photocoagulation, such as vitreous hemorrhage, are uncommon, but serous retinal detachment or aggravation of preexisting macular edema may occur. Perfused capillaries within the tumor indicate incomplete regression of an angioma. An excellent sign of regression is the development of a sclerotic feeding artery or reduced caliber of the feeding artery and draining vein. Repetition of treatment should be considered if the angioma has not regressed within 2 months. Pigment deposition within or adjacent to the angioma may allow improved absorption of additional photocoagulation to the tumor. Angiomas that progress or fail to regress in response to repeated photocoagulation may require external cryopexy.

TABLE 10–2. Parameters for Retinal Angioma Photocoagulation

Spot Size	200–500 μm
Burn Duration	0.2–0.5 sec
Initial Power Setting	180 mW
Wavelength	Dye yellow (577 nm) or argon green (514 nm)
Contact Lens	Rodenstock, three-mirror, or Goldmann
Anesthesia	Topical (≤ 1 DD) Retrobulbar (> 1 DD)

Goal: Treatment may be directed to the angioma surface, to the feeding artery, or to both structures. Confluent photocoagulation with a large spot size is applied when the angioma is treated directly. When the feeding artery is treated, the goal is to obtain a blanched tumor.

PRIMARY RETINAL TELANGIECTASIS (COATS' SYNDROME)

INTRODUCTION

Primary retinal telangiectasis, or Coats' syndrome, was first described in 1908.[19] Coats divided this syndrome into three categories (types) of patients based on funduscopic appearance. We now know that one category (Coats' type three) represented angiomatosis retinae. In 1912, Leber described patients with numerous small retinal capillary aneurysms (miliary aneurysms),[20] which he later realized exemplified Coats' type one.[21,22] In spite of Leber's clarification, many clinicians continued to discriminate between Coats' syndrome and Leber's miliary aneurysms. In 1956, Reese correctly observed that Leber's miliary aneurysms were indistinguishable from the spectrum of Coats' syndrome, and he originated the term "telangiectasis of the retina" to distinguish this form of exudative retinopathy.[23]

Most cases are not familial, although reports exist of involvement of multiple family members within a pedigree. The average age at diagnosis is 10 years, and 85 percent of cases appear in males. Most cases are unilateral.

Telangiectasia of the retinal vascular bed with an associated breakdown in the blood–retinal barrier is the fundamental abnormality seen in primary idiopathic retinal telangiectasis.[24,25] The telangiectatic vessel anomalies range from thickening of small vessel walls and slight dilation of the lumina to thinning of the vessel walls with loss of vascular endothelial cells and irregular dilation of the lumina. The early thickening of the capillary vessel walls is caused by deposition of excess basement membrane-like material admixed with accumulated lipid and plasma proteins. In advanced stages of the disease, all endothelial cells may be lost. The residual vessel walls consist of thickened, abnormal basement membrane-like material surrounded by glial cells. Ultimately, large areas of the vascular bed close, resulting in large areas of ischemic retina traversed by telangiectatic shunt vessels. Retinal and anterior segment neovascularization, vitreous hemorrhage, and neovascular glaucoma may then develop.[25]

DIAGNOSIS

Patient presentation in primary retinal telangiectasis is varied. Adult patients may (1) not have symptoms, (2) notice a moderate to mild decrease in central visual acuity and metamorphopsia due to retinal edema caused by exudation from leaking vessels, or (3) complain of a marked reduction in acuity due to compromised macular function. Advanced stages of the disease may be associated with uveitis, glaucoma, cataract, and phthisis bulbi. In small children, the diagnosis often is not made until the appearance of strabismus or leukokoria or the discovery on routine examination of an uncorrectable visual acuity deficit.

Primary retinal telangiectasis may be divided into five stages based on clinical severity.[25] One retinal quadrant is involved in 60 percent of these cases, and over 90 percent involve less than half the retinal area.[26] In more than two thirds of cases, the inferior temporal quadrant is affected. Because of the frequent involvement of the temporal quadrants, the macula is frequently compromised. Macular edema may be derived from telangiectatic vessels adjacent to the fovea (Fig. 10–2) or from peripheral vascular abnormalities.

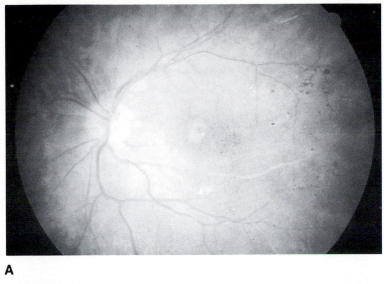

A

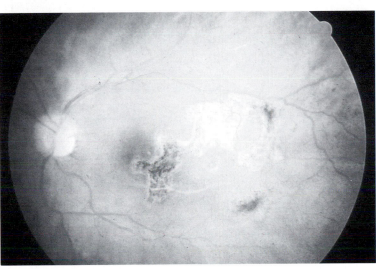

B

Figure 10–2. Stage one disease with telangiectatic vessels adjacent to the fovea (**A**) and after treatment with argon green laser (**B**).

Fundus fluorescein angiography is a useful diagnostic test in mild to moderate forms of the disease. Angiography also may be helpful in identifying areas to be treated. Hyperfluorescent light bulb-like lesions corresponding to aneurysmal dilation of vessels in the capillary bed, in association with leaking telangiectatic retinal vessels, are the most characteristic angiographic abnormality.[27] In addition, large areas of nonperfused retinal capillary bed may be seen. Moderate to severe leakage often occurs from the few remaining vessels. If the macula is adjacent to the area of involvement, the typical petaloid pattern of cystoid macular edema commonly is present. Large collections of yellow subretinal exudation, which may be found in advanced cases, may be hyperfluorescent or hypofluorescent presumably because of differences between cases in the rates of retinal vascular leakage.

The differential diagnosis of primary retinal telangiectasis in young patients includes retinoblastoma, retinopathy of prematurity, *Toxocara canis* infection, familial exudative vitreoretinopathy, angiomatosis retinae, and incontinentia pigmenti. Echography is useful in differentiating primary retinal telangiectasis from other causes of leukokoria, especially retinoblastoma. The typical B-scan pattern of retinoblastoma reveals a dome-shaped lesion, which by standardized A-scan is solid and contains extremely high reflective spikes, corresponding to focal calcification.[28] Calcification usually is not present in eyes with primary retinal telangiectasis.

LASER TREATMENT

Treatment Alternatives

The goal of treatment is to eliminate fluid exudation from the telangiectatic vessels and thereby reduce retinal edema and maintain apposition of the retina and choroid. Because telangiectatic vessel leakage progressively increases, treatment usually should be initiated on diagnosis. For therapy to be successful, all telangiectatic retinal vessels must be identified and treated. Unless excluded by an uncooperative young patient, a meticulous examination of the fundus with a three-mirror contact lens and a fluorescein angiogram of all visible retina should be performed to facilitate complete treatment. Intraoperative fluorescein angiography is sometimes useful in children because adequate preoperative examinations often are impossible.

Different therapeutic modalities may be required depending on disease severity (Table 10–3). Stage one disease should be treated with photocoagulation. Argon green is ideal because absorption of the green wavelength by the retinal pigment epithelium (RPE) produces sufficient damage to result in permanent closure of telangiectatic vessels (Fig. 10–2).

Stage two disease is more refractory to treatment than stage one because of the larger area of telangiectasis, accumulation of larger amounts of exudate, the loss of retinal transparency, and the thermal insulation between the retinal vessels and RPE due to accumulated subretinal exudate. Argon green photocoagulation has been shown effective in the treatment of this stage. Dye yellow (577 nm) also may be efficacious but has not been investigated adequately. Unresponsive lesions often require several photocoagulation sessions at 6-week intervals to eradicate sources of leakage. A combination of laser photocoagulation and cryopexy may be necessary to eradicate larger or more refractory telangiectatic vessels.

Stage three disease, characterized by a partial retinal detachment, and stage four disease, defined by a total retinal detachment, also may require photocoagulation or cryopexy or both to ablate exuding telangiectatic vessels. Multiple photocoagulation sessions usually are needed. When cryopexy is

TABLE 10–3. CLASSIFICATION OF STAGES OF SEVERITY OF PRIMARY RETINAL TELANGIECTASIS[a]

Stage one	Retinal telangiectasis
Stage two	Focal intraretinal exudates
Stage three	Partial retinal detachment
Stage four	Total retinal detachment
Stage five	Chronic retinal detachment

In stage one, most of the telangiectasis is confined to the capillary bed and there is minimal intraretinal exudation. In stage two there is more intraretinal exudation, cystoid macular edema, and circinate exudative maculopathy. In stages three and four, the exudate is present in the subretinal space, causing a partial or total retinal detachment. In stage five disease, there is retinal atrophy, which may be associated with subretinal membrane formation, chronic uveitis, neovascular glaucoma, cataract, or phthisis bulbi.

[a]After Sigelmann J: *Retinal Diseases: Pathogenesis, Laser Therapy and Surgery.* Boston: Little, Brown, and Co; 1984:332.

applied, transscleral drainage of subretinal fluid is necessary to reduce the scleral–retinal distance and allow adequate destruction (freezing) of telangiectatic vessels. Scleral buckling reduces the volume of the globe and may be helpful in some eyes with stage four disease. Retinal detachment portends a guarded prognosis, and visual recovery may be poor despite retinal reattachment.

Wavelength Selection

Argon green or blue-green wavelengths are useful in treating most cases. Dye yellow (577 nm) has not been evaluated adequately but has theoretical advantages over argon photocoagulation. Dye yellow, which is strongly absorbed by hemoglobin, may be more useful for occluding telangiectatic retinal vessels in detached retina.

Treatment Techniques

Many cases of primary retinal telangiectasia are diagnosed in children who will not tolerate unsedated fundus examination or treatment. General anesthesia may be required in this patient subgroup to facilitate treatment. Until recently, intraoperative external photocoagulation was not a widely accessible, easily performed modality. The indirect ophthalmoscopic laser delivery system allows young patients to receive photocoagulation in the supine position under general anesthesia.

Patients with localized disease in one or two quadrants who do not have extensive exudative detachment of the retina respond best to photocoagulation (Table 10–4). In the presence of extensive retinal detachment, argon green photocoagulation of the telangiectatic vessels can be attempted. However, this approach often fails because there is reduced heat transfer from the retinal pigment epithelium to the telangiectatic vessels. In these cases, vascular destruction may occur after direct vascular or intravascular hemoglobin absorption. Treatment with dye yellow may be attempted if an adequate treatment response is not obtained using argon green or blue-green.

Both photocoagulation and cryopexy lesions must induce intense vascular destruction and should cover all of the telangiectatic vessels, the intertelangiectatic shunt vessels, and microaneurysms adjacent to the involved areas.

TABLE 10–4. Parameters for Primary Retinal Telangiectasis (Coats' Syndrome) Photocoagulation

Spot Size	200–500 μm
Duration of Burn	0.2–0.5 sec
Initial Power Setting	150 mW
Wavelength	Argon green or dye yellow
Contact Lens	Goldmann or three-mirror
Anesthesia	Topical or retrobulbar

Goal: Lesions should be white and include all involved areas. Initial power setting of 150 mW will be inadequate if significant retinal edema exists, and laser power should be increased until white lesions are easily reproduced. Confluent photocoagulation burns should be placed over areas of moderate to marked vascular involvement. Small lesions near the fovea can be treated with individual or foci of closely spaced photocoagulation burns.

Follow-up and Complications

Complications after treatment of primary retinal telangiectasis are similar to those encountered in other retinal vascular diseases. Macular pucker occurs commonly in eyes that have been treated with both laser and cryopexy. Because photocoagulation close to the fovea often is required, the risk of a foveal burn is a frequent danger. Gass has reported total retinal detachment associated with proliferative vitreoretinopathy that occurred in an adult after peripheral cryopexy of telangiectatic vessels.[11] Other telangiectatic vessels may become apparent subsequent to treatment in affected individuals. Therefore, biannual or annual thorough fundus examinations should be performed throughout life.

IDIOPATHIC JUXTAFOVEAL RETINAL TELANGIECTASIS

INTRODUCTION

Idiopathic juxtafoveal retinal telangiectasis is an uncommon disease of the retinal capillaries in the foveal region that usually causes initial clinical symptoms during the fifth or sixth decade of life.[29] The etiology and pathogenesis of this disorder are not understood. It occurs with equal frequency in men and women and is usually bilateral. Telangiectatic retinal vessels with associated retinal edema or exudates usually are present in a localized one disc area or smaller region involving the temporal macula and fovea. Nasal macular involvement is less common.

DIAGNOSIS

Most patients with this disorder note metamorphopsia and a mild decrease in central visual acuity due to intraretinal edema derived from exuding retinal vessels. The visual acuity is typically 20/40 or better on initial symptomatic

---

TABLE 10–5. Parameters for Idiopathic Juxtafoveal Retinal Telangiectasis

Spot Size	50–100 μm
Duration of Burn	0.05–0.1 sec
Initial Power Setting	150 mW
Wavelength	Argon green
Contact Lens	Goldmann
Anesthesia	Topical or retrobulbar

Goal: Laser lesions of light to medium intensity are usually adequate. The lesions should be placed on the telangiectatic vessels and positioned 200 μm or more from the center of the fovea. After the initial treatment, the patient should be reevaluated at 8 or more weeks. If this initial treatment is not adequate, light applications should be repeated carefully. Laser treatment to choroidal neovascularization should be performed as described in Chapter 9.

---

examination. Most patients experience very slow deterioration of visual acuity over many years. Rarely will patients complain of rapid visual decline, a grave development that usually heralds the presence of a choroidal neovascular membrane compromising the fovea.

Funduscopic examination may reveal telangiectatic vessels with an associated blurring of the foveal reflex or grayish thickening of the fovea. In more advanced cases, examination may reveal cystoid macular edema, tiny deep intraretinal hemorrhages, microaneurysms, or yellowish white intraretinal exudation.

Fluorescein angiography confirms a mild dilation of the juxtafoveal capillaries, which fill during the early capillary phase and correspond to localized hyperfluorescence during the later phases. In some eyes, veins that extend at a right angle to the retinal surface and that drain the deep retinal plexus can be demonstrated by stereoscopic angiography.[29]

LASER TREATMENT

Treatment Techniques

Laser photocoagulation is the only treatment that has been demonstrated to successfully reduce macular edema, which complicates this disorder (Table 10–5). Treatment seldom is attempted for telangiectatic vessels with or without exudation because the involved vessels usually are adjacent to or involve the foveal capillary ring[11,29,30] and have a relatively benign prognosis. Extensive exudate with corresponding visual deterioration may indicate a need for photocoagulation.

In contrast, treatment should be considered immediately if a choroidal neovascular membrane develops. Choroidal neovascularization that develops in idiopathic juxtafoveal retinal telangiectasis often extends beneath the central fovea. Treatment in these cases should not be carried out. However, when choroidal neovascularization does not involve the center of the fovea, photocoagulation should be considered. Treatment guidelines for these cases are not well established, but reasonable initial laser parameters would be similar to those in patients with the presumed ocular histoplasmosis syndrome or idiopathic choroidal neovascularization.

Follow-up and Complications

If telangiectatic vessels have been treated, the fundus should be examined 8 weeks later to evaluate the effectiveness of the treatment. Because the leaking capillaries are usually so close to the center of the fovea, foveal damage is the major complication of treatment.

ACQUIRED RETINAL MACROANEURYSMS

INTRODUCTION

The term "retinal macroaneurysm" was first used in 1973 by Robertson[31] to distinguish fusiform or saccular retinal artery dilations, which typically occur within the first three bifurcations of the retinal arterial tree.[31] Other retinal vascular dilations, such as those associated with diabetes, vein occlusion, venous stasis due to carotid occlusions, and Coats' disease, were specifically not included.[31] These acquired lesions usually occur in patients during their sixth, seventh, or eighth decade of life.[31] Single macroaneurysms are most common, but multiple macroaneurysms may occur along the same retinal artery or elsewhere in the same eye.[32] Ten percent or fewer are found bilaterally.[32] The superotemporal artery is the most commonly reported site of involvement.[33,34] A large proportion of affected patients are female.[33] Systemic hypertension has been noted in one half to two thirds of patients harboring retinal macroaneurysms.[31-34]

DIAGNOSIS

The patient with a retinal macroaneurysm may be asymptomatic, concerned about deteriorating or compromised visual acuity from macroaneurysm-associated retinal edema or circinate exudation, or alarmed by a sudden visual loss due to macroaneurysm-associated hemorrhage. Fundus fluorescein angiography is the most useful diagnostic confirmatory test. Unless obscured by overlying hemorrhage, the aneurysm can be seen to fill during the retinal arterial phase. Aneurysm wall leakage progresses throughout the venous and late angiographic phases. Other abnormalities that may be seen within the adjacent capillary bed include microaneurysm formation and capillary dilation. In some cases, the affected retinal artery may demonstrate vascular caliber irregularity, a delay in filling, or both.

The natural course of an individual retinal macroaneurysm is unpredictable.[33-35] Incipient arterial dilations may be noted, which typically occur at arteriovenous crossings or at artery bifurcations (Fig. 10–3). Occasionally, intraluminal emboli may be seen within the macroaneurysm or at other arterial bifurcations.[32,34] Pulsatile macroaneurysms also have been observed.[32] Macroaneurysms may involute or may decompensate, thereby producing adjacent or distant foveal retinal edema. Intraretinal hemorrhage resulting from a macroaneurysm may remain sequestered beneath the internal limiting membrane within the neurosensory retina or may extend into the preretinal, vitreous, or subretinal space. Because hemorrhage may obscure the bleeding site and may occur within a variety of tissue spaces, these patients frequently receive an incorrect diagnosis.[36] Based on natural history studies, retinal macroaneurysms have been divided into three groups[33]: (A) macroaneurysms in which the edema, exudate, or hemorrhage is located within the temporal arcades, resulting in decreased visual acuity at presentation, (B) those in which edema, exudate, or hemorrhage is located within the macula without compromise of visual acuity, and (C) macroaneurysms with associated edema, exudate, or hemorrhage confined to the extramacular retina. Most macroaneurysms spontaneously involute without substantially affecting visual acuity.[31] Patients who have suffered previous central visual loss (group A) or those in whom the macroaneurysm affects the extramacular retina (group C) are unlikely to benefit from laser photocoagulation. Photocoagulation, however, may speed visual recovery or prevent visual loss in those macroaneurysms in which associated retinal edema involves or threatens the fovea (group B).[33-35] Extensive macroaneurysm-associated hemorrhage is a relative contraindication to photocoagulation because many of these macroaneurysms demonstrate a subsequent spontaneous reduction in retinal edema, exudate, or both.

LASER TREATMENT

The primary goal of treatment should be to reduce the macroaneurysm-associated macular edema that compromises or imminently threatens the fovea. Treatment should be directed to the incompetent retinal capillaries sur-

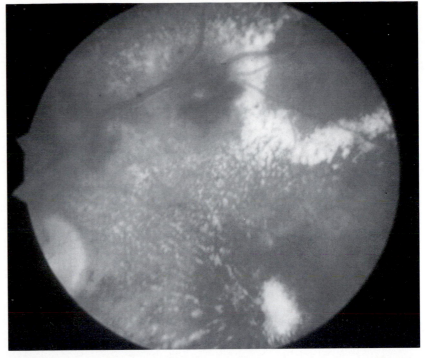

A

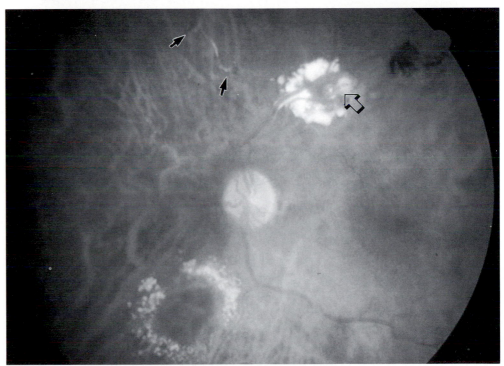

B

Figure 10–3. Sequential fundus photographs depicting multiple untreated retinal arterial macroaneurysms in a variety of stages. **A.** This 57-year-old hypertensive male had a visual acuity of 20/200 when first seen. **B.** Note the regression of macular exudate and resolution of the macular star as the retinal edema spontaneously resolves over the next 6 years. The superotemporal macroaneurysm is seen as a fibrotic white nodule (*large arrow*). A spontaneously occluded macroaneurysm and proximal sclerotic artery are also present (*small arrows*). (*Photographs courtesy of Sohan S. Hayreh, M.D., Ph.D., University of Iowa.*)

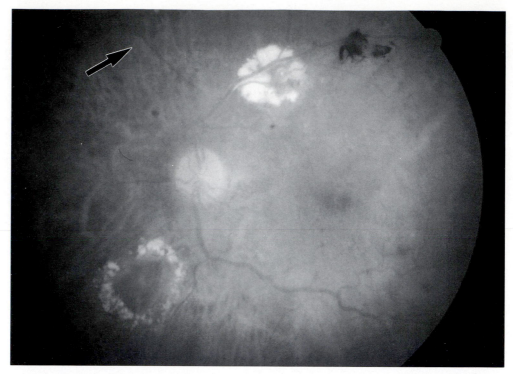

C

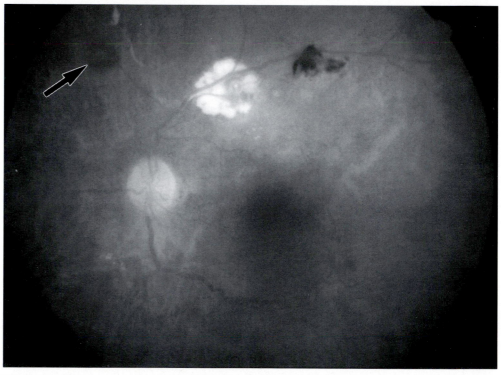

D

Figure 10–3 (Continued). Subsequent photographs taken 15 (**C**) and 23 (**D**) months later show the progression from an incipient lesion to a new macroaneurysm (*arrows*). Photocoagulation, if performed after central visual loss has occurred, may be of no benefit if the visual loss is long standing and retains the risk of branch retinal artery occlusion. *(Photographs courtesy of Sohan S. Hayreh, M.D., Ph.D., University of Iowa.)*

rounding macroaneurysms[33] and, perhaps, to the macroaneurysm wall. Care should be taken to avoid treatment directly over the retinal artery. Though not well studied, lowering systemic hypertension should not be neglected in those patients who demonstrate increased diastolic or systolic blood pressure on presentation to the ophthalmologist. Consultation for management of hypertension may be indicated.

Wavelength Selection

Recently, lasers emitting wavelengths strongly absorbed by hemoglobin, such as dye yellow (577 nm), have been advocated for the treatment of macular edema resulting from retinal arterial macroaneurysms.[17,37,38] Assuming that the photocoagulation effects are due to intraluminal hemoglobin absorption adjacent to the macroaneurysm wall or within the incompetent capillary lumina, hemoglobin-absorbing wavelengths would be expected to deliver an increased fraction of energy to the desired target. In particular, surgeons should avoid the use of dye yellow wavelength when photocoagulating macroaneurysms associated with intraretinal hemorrhage because of the risk of branch retinal artery occlusion distal to the macroaneurysm.[39] Branch retinal artery occlusion may occur shortly after photocoagulation of the macroaneurysm[39] and may go unnoticed.[38,40] The argon green (514 nm) wavelength is probably safer than dye yellow for treating macroaneurysms that are proximal to arteries that feed the macula or are adjacent to retinal hemorrhage.

Treatment Techniques

After obtaining informed consent, which should include a discussion of the possible risks of photocoagulation-induced hemorrhage and branch retinal artery occlusion, topical anesthesia is instilled into the fornix. Rarely is retrobulbar anesthetic required. Dye yellow photocoagulation is the preferred wavelength if associated intraretinal hemorrhage is not present. Argon green (514 nm) is preferred when associated hemorrhage is present and is an acceptable alternative to dye yellow. A spot size of 200 to 500 μm allows adequate photocoagulation with a minimum of laser power. A suitable burn can usually be obtained at 0.1 sec, but this may be increased to 0.2 or 0.5 sec as needed to obtain sufficient burn intensity (Table 10–6). The initial power setting should be as low as the dye laser will allow, typically 100 mW. Contact lens preferences vary from surgeon to surgeon. The authors prefer the Goldmann or three-mirror fundus lens.

TABLE 10–6. Parameters for Macroaneurysm Photocoagulation

Spot Size	200–500 μm
Duration of Burn	0.1–0.5 sec
Initial Power Setting	100 mW
Wavelength	Dye yellow (577 nm) or argon green (574 nm)
Contact Lens	Goldmann or three-mirror
Anesthesia	Topical

Goal: The edge of the macroaneurysm is treated with moderately white laser burns, avoiding the afferent and efferent artery. Larger, lower intensity burns can be placed over the macroaneurysm wall to obtain a light blanching effect.

Follow-up and Complications

Patients should be seen within 3 weeks after photocoagulation to evaluate patency of the artery in the distribution of the macroaneurysm. Intraretinal exudate may require months or years to regress. Intraretinal macular edema may respond much more quickly and can be monitored by Hruby or Goldmann contact lens examination. If visual deterioration occurs, repeat fluorescein angiography is advisable. A Goldmann visual field also may be helpful if a branch retinal artery occlusion is suspected.[40] Repeat photocoagulation may be considered if after several months there is no evidence of reduced retinal edema or exudate or if there is an increase in macular edema that correlates with a decrease in central visual acuity.

CHOROIDAL HEMANGIOMA

INTRODUCTION

A cavernous hemangioma of the choroid is a benign, idiopathic hamartoma composed of widely dilated, thin-walled, endothelium-lined vascular channels with little intervening connective tissue. They may be associated with Sturge-Weber syndrome, in which they typically cause a slight or moderate diffuse elevation of the involved choroid, or choroidal hemangiomas may exist as isolated localized tumors in patients with no other vascular malformations.[41,42] Isolated hemangiomas usually are elevated lesions that can occur anywhere in the posterior pole of the eye. However, they have a predilection for the area around the macula. Tumor growth is probably maximal during the physiologic growth period, with a typical isolated lesion reaching 3 to 30 mm in diameter when first seen.[11] They are seldom symptomatic before the third decade of life.

DIAGNOSIS

The first clinical symptom usually is blurred or distorted vision. Flashes of light and floaters are sometimes prominent. Visual compromise probably results from cystic and other degenerative changes in the sensory retina overlying the tumor. There may be a serous detachment of the macular area caused by leakage of serous fluid from the incompetent walls of the sinuses of the tumor. As the cystic retinal degeneration and serous detachment of the central retina become chronic, a profound loss of central vision, increasing hyperopia, and an enlarging scotoma may develop. Serous detachment separating the retina from the entire tumor surface is uncommon, but occasionally a localized bullous or very extensive detachment with complete loss of formed vision may occur.[11]

The appearance of isolated choroidal hemangiomas depends on the duration the tumor has been present, the degree of retinal pigment epithelial alteration, and the degree of associated glial proliferation. If seen before secondary changes have occurred, the tumor is a localized, dome-shaped, orange-colored mass. The overlying retina, which may be detached, initially appears whitish in color but, after a prolonged period, may become atrophic or so markedly pigmented it obscures the tumor. The choroidal hemangioma surface may develop a white, red, brown, or green color. Occasionally, because of associated hyperplasia of the overlying retinal pigment epithelium, these tumors are confused with pigmented malignant melanomas.[11]

Fluorescein angiography usually reveals marked early hyperfluorescence of the large sinusoidal (choroidal) vascular channels during the prearterial and arterial phases.[43] Venous and later phases of the angiogram may reveal a ring of hypofluorescence corresponding to the peripheral part of the hemangioma.[44] After the early phases, there is widespread leakage from these sinusoidal vessels that account for much of the tumor. Choroidal leakage often accumulates in the outer retina, resulting in a diffuse polycystic pattern during late phases of the angiogram. Eyes with marked thickening and whitening of the retina may demonstrate only a diffuse choroidal hyperfluorescence during the early phases.

Standardized A-scan echography is very useful in differentiating a choroidal hemangioma from malignant melanoma, metastatic tumor, or other solitary lesions. The typical standardized A-scan pattern reveals a solid, highly reflective lesion that contains a series of congruent repeating spikes.[45] Separation between the retinal reflection and the lesion surface indicates that there may be an associated retinal detachment. The blood flow is so sluggish through the cavernous vessel luminae that no detectable variation in vessel caliber is detectable echographically.

The differential diagnosis of orange-colored tumors of the fundus includes metastatic carcinoma, amelanotic melanoma, choroidal osteoma, nodular scleritis, and retinal capillary hemangioma.[11]

LASER TREATMENT

Treatment Alternatives

Photocoagulation or cryopexy can be used alone or may be combined to treat choroidal hemangiomas depending on the location and size of the tumor.[46,47] Isolated tumors that are not causing retinal detachment or retinal degeneration do not need treatment.[41] Tumors located in the posterior pole are most easily treated by laser, whereas those located in the anterior fundus are most easily treated by cryopexy. Some eyes in patients who have the Sturge-Weber syndrome have such extensive involvement and the required treatment area is so great that much of the eye would be destroyed. Tumors contiguous with the optic nerve or fovea may be treated with photocoagulation, but cryopexy should not be used to avoid injury to these vital structures.

Wavelength Selection

Argon green and blue-green wavelengths have been used to photocoagulate choroidal hemangiomas. Dye yellow photocoagulation may have some use and may be tried if argon green or blue-green wavelengths are not effective.

Treatment Techniques

It is difficult if not impossible to occlude the dilated sinusoidal choroidal vessels. The goal of treatment is to reduce leakage from the vessels by applying light to medium intensity laser burns over the tumor surface (Table 10–7). Large lesions, from 300 to 1000 μm spot size, are preferred. Medium intensity burns are placed contiguously over the entire lesion (Fig. 10–4), and repeated treatments often are necessary to reduce or eliminate exudation. Small lesions can be treated with topical anesthesia, but larger lesions require retrobulbar anesthesia to control pain.

Follow-up and Complications

Paradoxically, treatment may increase choroidal vascular leakage. Lamellar macular holes, chronic cystoid macular edema, and epiretinal membranes may occur. Excessive treatment may lead to extensive chorioretinal scarring, retinal

TABLE 10–7. Parameters for Choroidal Cavernous Hemangioma Photocoagulation

Spot Size	300–1000 μm
Duration of Burn	0.2–0.5 sec
Initial Power Setting	150 mW
Wavelength	Argon green or argon blue-green or dye yellow
Contact Lens	Goldmann or Rodenstock or three-mirror
Anesthesia	Topical or retrobulbar

Goal: Laser lesions of light to medium intensity usually are adequate. Treatment should cover the entire tumor with contiguous laser lesions.

hole formation, ruptured choroidal vessels, massive choroidal hemorrhage, and other complications. Patients should be evaluated 6 to 8 weeks after treatment. Adequate treatment may be assessed by reduction of retinal edema, reduction of associated serous retinal detachment, or improvement in visual acuity. If this initial treatment is inadequate, carefully repeat light applications of additional photocoagulation burns and repeat fundus examination after 8 weeks. Successfully treated patients should be reexamined at 6- to 12-month intervals.

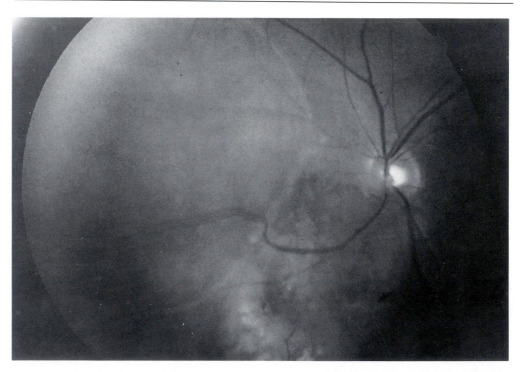

Figure 10–4A. Choroidal cavernous hemangioma nasal to the disc. Note the associated bullous, nonrhegmatogenous retinal detachment extending from the nasal aspect of the choroidal hemangioma.

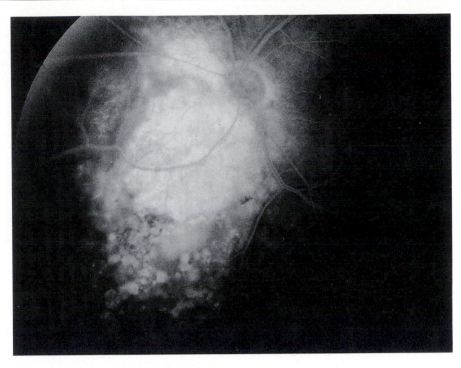

Figure 10–4B. Late-phase fluorescein angiogram demonstrating the hyperfluorescence from the choroidal hemangioma.

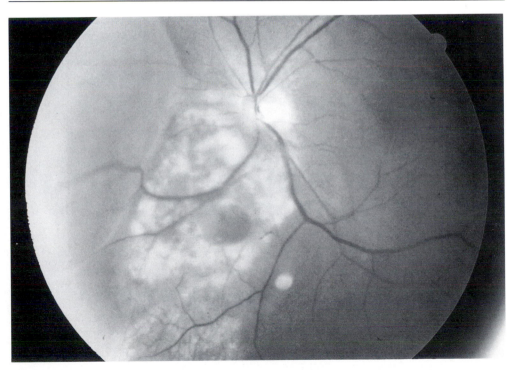

Figure 10–4C. Immediately after dye yellow laser treatment. Confluent 500 μm, low-intensity, laser burns of 0.5 to 1.0 sec duration were used to cover the surface of the hemangioma.

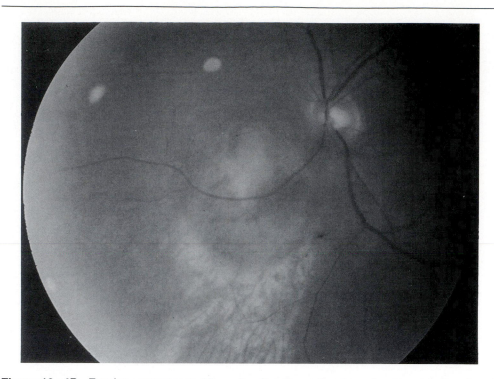

Figure 10–4D. Fundus appearance 10 weeks after dye yellow laser treatment to the choroidal hemangioma. Note the complete resolution of the associated retinal detachment. The choroidal hemangioma appears relatively unchanged.

REFERENCES

1. von Hippel E: Uber eine sehr seltene Erkrankung der Netzhaut. *Arch Ophthalmol* 1904:59:83–106.
2. Lindau A: Zur frage der angiomatosis retinae und ihrer hirnkomplikationen. *Acta Ophthalmol* 1927;4:193–226.
3. Watzke RC, Weingeist TA, Constantine JB: Diagnosis and management of von Hippel-Lindau disease. In: Peyman GA, Apple DJ, Sanders DR, eds. *Intraocular Tumors*. New York: Appleton-Century-Crofts; 1977:199–217.
4. Seizinger BR, Rouleau GA, Ozelius LJ, Lane AH, Farmer GE, Lamiell JM, Haines J, Yuen JWM, Collins D, Majoor-Krakauer D, Bonner T, Mathew C, Rubenstein A, Halperin J, McConkie-Rosell A, Green JS, Trofatter JA, Ponder BA, Eierman L, Bowmer MI, Schimke R, Oostra B, Aronin N, Smith DI, Drabkin H, Waziri MH, Hobbs WJ, Martuza RL, Conneally PM, Hsia YE, Gusella JF: von Hippel-Lindau disease maps to the region of chromosome 3 associated with renal cell carcinoma. *Nature* 1988;332:268–269.
5. McKusick VA: *Mendelian Inheritance in Man: Catalogs of Autosomal Dominant, Autosomal Recessive, and X-linked Phenotypes*, 8th ed. Baltimore: Johns Hopkins University Press; 1988.
6. Ridley M, Green J, Johnson G: Retinal angiomatosis: the ocular manifestations of von Hippel-Lindau disease. *Can J Ophthalmol* 1986;21:276–283.
7. Lowden BA, Harris GS: Pheochromocytoma and von Hippel-Lindau disease. *Can J Ophthalmol* 1976;11:282–289.
8. Jesberg DO, Spencer WH, Hoyt WF: Incipient lesions of von Hippel-Lindau disease. *Arch Ophthalmol* 1968;80:632–640.
9. Lane CM, Turner G, Gregor ZJ, Bird AC: Laser treatment of retinal angiomatosis. *Eye* 1989;3:33–38.
10. Nicholson DH, Anderson LS, Blodi C: Rhegmatogenous retinal detachment in angiomatosis retinae. *Am J Ophthalmol* 1986;101:187–189.

11. Gass JDM: *Stereoscopic Atlas of Macular Disease: diagnosis and treatment*, 3rd ed. St. Louis, MO: CV Mosby Co; 1987.
12. Gass JDM: Treatment of retinal vascular anomalies. *Ophthalmology* 1977;83:OP432–442.
13. Annesley WH, Leonard BC, Shields JA, Tasman WS: Fifteen year review of treated cases of retinal angiomatosis. *Ophthalmology* 1977;83:OP446–453.
14. Peyman GA, Redman KRV, Mottow-Lippa L, Flood T: Treatment of large von Hippel tumors by eye wall resection. *Ophthalmology* 1983;90:840–847.
15. Cardosa RD, Brockhurst RJ: Penetrating diathermy coagulation for retinal angiomas. *Arch Ophthalmol* 1976;94:1702–1715.
16. Nicholson DH: Induced ocular hypertension during photocoagulation of afferent artery in angiomatosis retinae. *Retina* 1983;3:59–61.
17. Folk JC, Russell SR: Appropriate wavelength for posterior segment laser photocoagulation. American Academy of Ophthalmology, *Focal Points 1988: Clinical Modules for Ophthalmologists*, Module 7, 1988.
18. Blodi CF, Russell SR, Pulido JS, Folk JC: Direct and feeder vessel photocoagulation of retinal angiomas with dye yellow laser. *Ophthalmology* 1990;97:791–797.
19. Coats G: Forms of retinal disease with massive exudation. *R Lond Ophthalmic Hosp Rep* 1908;17:440–525.
20. Leber TH: Uber eine durch Vorkommen multipler Miliaraneurysmen charakterisierte Form von Retinaldegeneration. *Graefe's Arch Ophthalmol* 1912;81:1–14.
21. Leber TH: Die Aneurysmen der Zentralarterie und ihrer Verzweigungen: Retinaldegeneration bei multiplen Miliaraneurysmen. *Graefe-Saemisch Handbuch der Augenheilkunde* 1915;7:20–36.
22. Leber TH: Die Retinitis exsudativa (Coats), Retinitis und Chorioretinitis serofibrinosa degenerans. *Graefe-Saemisch Handbuch der Augenheilkunde* 1916;7:1267–1319.
23. Reese AB: Telangiectasis of the retina and Coats' disease. *Am J Ophthalmol* 1956;42:1–8.
24. Manschot WA, Bruijyn WC: Coats' disease: definition and pathogenesis. *Br J Ophthalmol* 1967;51:145–157.
25. Sigelmann J: *Retinal Diseases: Pathogenesis, Laser Therapy and Surgery.* Boston: Little, Brown, and Co; 1984:332.
26. Fox KR: Coats' disease. *Metabol Pediatr Ophthalmol* 1980;4:121–124.
27. Gass JDM: A fluorescein angiographic study of macular dysfunction secondary to retinal vascular disease: V. Retinal telangiectasis. *Arch Ophthalmol* 1968;80:592–617.
28. Hermsen VM: Echographic diagnosis. In: Blodi FC, ed. *Retinoblastoma.* New York: Churchill Livingstone; 1985:111–127.
29. Gass JDM, Oyakawa RT: Idiopathic juxtafoveolar retinal telangiectasis. *Arch Ophthalmol* 1982;100:769–780.
30. Chopdar A: Retinal telangiectasis in adults: fluorescein angiographic findings and treatment by argon laser. *Br J Ophthalmol* 1978;62:243–250.
31. Robertson DM: Macroaneurysms of the retinal arteries. *Trans Am Acad Ophthalmol Otolaryngol* 1973;77:OP55–67.
32. Gass JDM: *Stereoscopic Atlas of Macular Diseases: Diagnosis and Treatment*, 2nd ed. St. Louis, MO: CV Mosby Co; 1977.
33. Palastine AG, Robertson DM, Goldstein BG: Macroaneurysms of the retinal arteries. *Am J Ophthalmol* 1982;93:164–171.
34. Lewis RA, Norton EWD, Gass JDM: Acquired arterial macroaneurysms of the retina. *Br J Ophthalmol* 1976;60:21–30.
35. Abdel-Khalek MN, Richardson J: Retinal macroaneurysm: natural history and guidelines for treatment. *Br J Ophthalmol* 1986;70:2–11.
36. Irvine AR: The diagnoses most commonly missed by ophthalmologists referring patients for fluorescein angiography. *Ophthalmology* 1986;93:1216–1221.
37. Mainster MA, Whitacre MM: Dye yellow photocoagulation of retinal arterial macroaneurysms. *Am J Ophthalmol* 1988;105:97–98.
38. Joondeph BC, Joondeph HC, Blair NP: Retinal macroaneurysms treated with the yellow dye laser. *Retina* 1989;9:187–192.
39. Russell SR, Folk JC: Branch retinal artery occlusion after dye yellow photocoagulation of an arterial macroaneurysm. *Am J Ophthalmol* 1987;104:186–187.
40. Russell SR: Letter to the editor. *Retina* 1990;10:229.
41. Gass DJM: *Differential Diagnosis of Intraocular Tumors: A Stereoscopic Presentation.* St.

Louis, MO: CV Mosby Co; 1974:113–138.

42. Witschel H, Font RL: Hemangioma of the choroid: a clinicopathologic study of 71 cases and a review of the literature. *Surv Ophthalmol* 1976;20:415–431.

43. Norton EWD, Gutman F: Fluorescein angiography and hemangiomas of the choroid. *Arch Ophthalmol* 1967;78:121–125.

44. Gass JDM: Photocoagulation of macular lesions. *Trans Am Acad Ophthalmol Otolaryngol* 1971;75:580–608.

45. Ossoinig KC, Blodi FC: Preoperative differential diagnosis of tumors with echography: III. Diagnosis of intraocular tumors. In: Blodi FC, ed. *Current Concepts in Ophthalmology*. St. Louis, MO: CV Mosby Co; 1974;4:296.

46. Humphrey WT: Choroidal hemangioma: response to cryotherapy. *Ann Ophthalmol* 1979;11:100–104.

47. Sanborn GE, Augsburger JJ, Shields JA: Treatment of circumscribed choroidal hemangiomas. *Ophthalmology* 1982;89:1374–1380.

CHAPTER 11

Retinal Breaks

Patrick J. Caskey and Patrick Coonan

INTRODUCTION

Retinal breaks are quite common, occurring in 3 to 7 percent of the adult population in clinical series, and are asymptomatic in most cases.[1-3] However, a small percentage (1–2 percent) of patients with retinal breaks will progress to retinal detachment.[1,4] The management of retinal breaks with laser requires an understanding of the natural history of a retinal tear, the risk factors known to predispose to retinal detachment, and the alternatives for treatment.

NATURAL HISTORY AND DIAGNOSIS

Throughout life, the vitreous undergoes a gradual morphologic evolution. In infancy and childhood, the vitreous is a homogeneous gel-like matrix of water, collagen fibrils, and hyaluronates that occupies the ocular volume between the retina and crystalline lens.[5] The entire retina is in contact with the vitreous in this age group.[6] As the individual matures, the vitreous begins to break down into a composite of gel matrix and fluid pockets in a process known as syneresis.[7,8] With continued liquefaction, this syneretic vitreous begins to separate from the inner limiting membrane of the retina and coalesces into the midvitreous,[8] a process that often results in entopic phenomena (visible floaters) and photopias (light flashes). In most cases, vitreous separation occurs atraumatically, progressing anteriorly to terminate eventually at the vitreous base.

Retinal tears occur as this normal separation of the posterior vitreous encounters an area of excessive vitreoretinal adhesion. These areas are most commonly located at the posterior margin of the anterior vitreous base, where vitreous collagen fibers firmly insert into the basement membrane of the Müller cells of the retina.[9] When the advancing line of vitreous separation impinges on such an adhesion, traction between the vitreous and retina develops. Eventually, as this traction increases, either the vitreous pulls free of the retina, leaving the retina intact, or the retina tears. If a tear occurs, the torn retina may continue to pull entirely free from the underlying retinal pigment epithelium (RPE), releasing the vitreoretinal traction and resulting in a retinal operculum suspended within the vitreous.

Often, however, the tear does not pull free but continues to enlarge due to persistent traction. This results in the occurrence of a typical horseshoe-shaped flap retinal tear. This full-thickness break creates a conduit for the passage of liquid vitreous under the retina. The resulting accumulation of subretinal fluid may produce widespread detachment of the retina from the RPE.

A variety of ocular entities are associated with an increased incidence of retinal tear formation. Lattice degeneration appears in 8 to 10 percent of the population[10,11] and comprises areas of retinal thinning associated with increased vitreoretinal traction. This combination results in a predisposition for retinal breaks and detachment, and up to 35 percent of all retinal detachments are associated with lattice lesions.[12]

High or progressive myopia (greater than 6.00 D) is another risk factor for the formation of retinal breaks.[13] The anteroposterior elongation of the globe noted in highly myopic patients results in stretching and thinning of the peripheral retina, which increases the potential for retinal tearing as the vitreous separates. High myopia and lattice degeneration often occur concurrently,[14] possibly producing a higher incidence of retinal breaks than either entity individually.

Atrophic, full-thickness retinal holes commonly are seen in the general population, often within regions of lattice degeneration.[10,15] They are associated with retinal detachment relatively infrequently.[16] However, if an atrophic hole has appreciable surrounding subretinal fluid or is associated with increased vitreoretinal traction, the potential for retinal detachment may be greater.

Aphakic and pseudophakic patients also are at increased risk for the development of retinal breaks.[17,18] All available techniques used at present for lensectomy unavoidably result in some degree of vitreous movement, with secondary tractional forces exerted at the ora serrata and at regions of excessive vitreoretinal adhesion. This vitreous manipulation may cause minute retinal breaks that can remain asymptomatic for extended periods after cataract surgery. Later, as vitreous fluid passes through the break, the patient may manifest a symptomatic retinal detachment. Retinal detachment occurs in up to 5 percent of aphakic and pseudophakic patients after intracapsular cataract extraction.[17] As extracapsular techniques have become the standard of care, the incidence of detachment has declined to less than 2 percent.[18]

Other predisposing factors for retinal break formation are less common and include blunt trauma,[19] regressed retinopathy of prematurity,[20] retinal infection (Cytomegalovirus, acute retinal necrosis, endophthalmitis),[21-23] and a variety of hereditary disorders (Stickler syndrome, X-linked retinoschisis, Marfan syndrome, Goldmann-Favre syndrome).[24]

LASER TREATMENT

Treatment Alternatives

Laser photocoagulation and transscleral cryopexy both have been used successfully and extensively for treatment of retinal breaks. Specific advantages of laser photocoagulation over cryopexy have been identified in recent years, and this modality has become the treatment of choice in most clinical settings. Laser photocoagulation appears to result in less inflammation than cryopexy, which may reduce the incidence of proliferative vitreoretinopathy. Laser photocoagulation has been shown to result in less breakdown of the blood–retinal barrier and less release of chemoattractants for RPE cells.[25,26] Because scleral indentation is not required, laser photocoagulation also may result in less dispersion of RPE cells into the vitreous than does cryopexy.[27] An adequate chorioretinal adhesion from cryopexy is reported to require up to 10 days for completion,[28,29] whereas a firm adhesion from laser photocoagulation has been demonstrated after 24 hours (Fig. 11–1).[30,31]

Despite the advantages of laser photocoagulation, some retinal breaks may be treated more effectively by cryopexy. Laser energy delivered through a contact lens may not effectively reach very anterior breaks. This location results in easy access for the cryoprobe, and peripheral tears and dialyses traditionally have been treated in this fashion. With the advent of the binocular indirect laser, however, most of these peripheral breaks can now be treated adequately with the laser (see Chapter 17). In patients in whom significant vitreous hemorrhage has occurred, diffusion of light may hinder visualization of the break and prevent laser energy from producing an effective photocoagulation burn. In these cases, placing the patient at bedrest with elevation of the head for several hours often will result in enough clearing to allow successful laser treatment. If the vitreous hemorrhage fails to clear sufficiently, cryopexy often can still be administered if the view of the break allows for assessment of the location and adequacy of treatment.

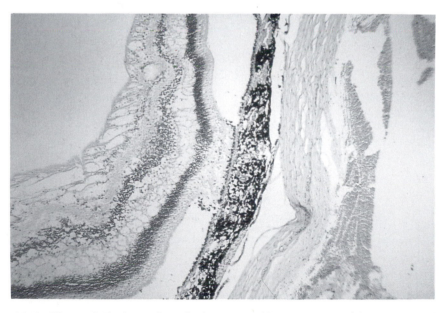

Figure 11–1. Histopathologic section of a krypton red laser burn placed in the eye of cynomolgus monkey 24 hours before fixation. The retina is artifactitiously detached except at the treatment site. Hematoxylineosin. ×50.4 (original magnification).

Goals of Laser Treatment

Laser treatment is used to seal the break by creating an adhesion between the surrounding retinal tissue and underlying RPE. This provides a barrier to continued enlargement of the tear from persistent vitreoretinal traction and prevents the accumulation of subretinal fluid at the tear site by limiting the potential flow of liquid vitreous through the tear. Subretinal fluid adjacent to the tear may be effectively contained within the encircling treatment ring, preventing the formation of more extensive detachment.

This adhesion is formed as light energy from the laser is absorbed by the pigmented cells within the RPE. Thermal conversion then results in heat production, which causes coagulation of the adjacent retinal, RPE, and choroidal tissues. As previously mentioned, this coagulative process has been demonstrated to produce a firm chorioretinal adhesion within 24 hours, and the strength of the adhesion probably continues to increase over several days. By linking individual laser burns, the encircling barrier around the retinal break can be effectively custom-fit for each retinal tear.

Indications for Treatment

Risk factors predisposing to retinal detachment in patients with retinal breaks have been identified and may be summarized in a treatment algorithm (Fig. 11–2). Before laser intervention, a careful ophthalmoscopic appraisal of the location and number of potentially treatable retinal lesions should be made. A cursory examination may result in breaks that are treated inadequately or missed entirely and is a common cause of treatment failure.

Once the extent of the retinal pathologic condition has been determined, the decision to treat is based on several parameters. The type of retinal lesion is an important consideration. Full-thickness flap tears (with or without associated lattice degeneration) are more likely to result in retinal detachment than are atrophic holes, vitreoretinal traction tufts, or isolated regions of lattice

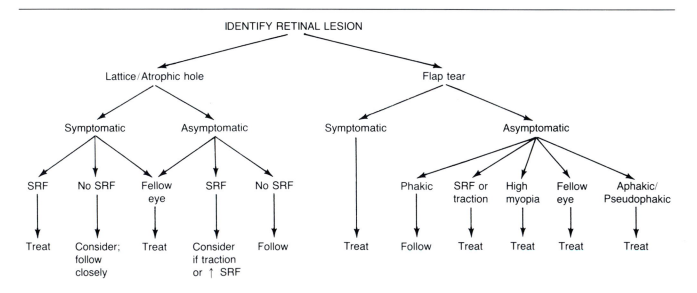

*Consider treating tractional tufts if symptomatic and associated with increasing traction and/or adjacent hemorrhage.

*Consider early prophylactic treatment for superior lesions and follow any nontreated superior lesions carefully.

*Treat lattice, holes or tears prophylactically at least 2 weeks before intraocular surgery, YAG capsulotomy, or initiating miotic therapy for glaucoma.

Figure 11–2. Basic guidelines for management of retinal breaks and lattice degeneration.

without breaks. Most full-thickness tears should, therefore, be considered for treatment. Atrophic holes, traction tufts, and simple lattice are not ordinarily treated unless other factors are present that suggest an increased potential for retinal detachment formation.

Acute symptoms (i.e., photopsia and entopic phenomena) are usually an indication of recent vitreous separation, with potential tractional damage to the retina. Photopsias generally are thought to be caused by stimulation of retinal photoreceptors by active vitreoretinal traction. Entopic phenomena represent the patient's subjective visual awareness of coalescent vitreous debris or hemorrhage produced as the vitreous pulls free of the retina. These symptoms are associated with an increased risk of eventual break enlargement and retinal detachment. Therefore, any flap tear associated with acute symptoms within the previous few weeks should undergo treatment.

Symptomatic patients with only atrophic holes or simple lattice commonly are treated prophylactically but often will progress to complete posterior vitreous separation in a benign fashion without laser intervention. If the decision not to treat is made, however, close follow-up (at least weekly) is critical, and laser photocoagulation should be administered immediately if the lesion becomes associated with subretinal fluid (implying a new full-thickness tear) or there is evidence of increasing traction. Symptomatic tractional tufts should be monitored carefully for the presence of adjacent intraretinal hemorrhage, which often precedes formation of a flap tear. Treatment should be initiated as soon as the hemorrhage is discovered to prevent flap tear evolution.

Atrophic holes and lattice lesions often are discovered during routine evaluation of the peripheral retina. These asymptomatic lesions typically are long standing in nature and have little tendency to result in more extensive retinal damage. Accordingly, these patients may be managed by routine follow-up, and laser treatment usually is not indicated. However, the presence of excessive vitreoretinal traction or subclinical detachment (subretinal fluid up to 2 disc areas in extent) may suggest a less benign course, and prophylactic laser photocoagulation should be considered. If the lesion is located superiorly, greater emphasis should be placed on laser intervention, since the macula may be placed at increased risk of detachment due to downward gravitational shift of accumulating subretinal fluid.

Asymptomatic full-thickness tears are relatively common in normal phakic eyes. These tend to remain stable, especially if associated with surrounding pigment demarcation, and do not require laser treatment in the majority of cases. Yearly fundus examination usually is sufficient for follow-up unless special circumstances are present that appreciably increase the risk of retinal detachment. As with atrophic holes and lattice degeneration, the presence of subclinical retinal detachment or increased vitreoretinal traction increases this risk and argues for laser intervention, particularly if the tear is located superiorly. Patients with high myopia and asymptomatic tears may exhibit an increased probability of progression to retinal detachment, and laser treatment appears warranted in this situation.

Any lattice lesions, atrophic holes, or flap tears in the fellow eye of a patient with a previous retinal detachment should be considered for treatment whether symptomatic or not. These patients have demonstrated a tendency for detachment to occur in one eye and may be at higher risk for detachment in the fellow eye. Prophylactic laser treatment appears to be indicated in the majority of these cases.

Aphakic and pseudophakic eyes with full-thickness breaks represent a special situation where two risk factors for retinal detachment coexist. Laser treatment should be administered to all flap tears in this setting, since the additive risk of the previous surgical vitreous manipulation and the tear itself probably results in a higher potential for retinal detachment.

If anticipating procedures that may result in acute vitreous shift with traction, such as intraocular surgery, YAG capsulotomy, or initiation of miotic therapy for glaucoma, prophylactic treatment of all holes, tears, and lattice lesions should be considered to lessen the potential for detachment. Treatment should be scheduled at least 2 weeks before the planned procedure to allow the laser adhesion to mature fully.

Wavelength Selection

Of the variety of laser wavelengths available for use within the eye, those that exhibit uptake by the pigment of the RPE have the greatest clinical use for treatment of breaks. This characteristic allows for production of heat at the interface between the retina and the RPE, which in turn results in efficient coagulation and adhesion formation. The green wavelength (414.5 nm) of the argon laser is effectively absorbed by the RPE and is the wavelength used most frequently for retinal break treatment. The argon blue component (488.0 nm) is absorbed by the RPE but also is absorbed by the vitreous and may produce heating with vitreous contraction. The xanthochrome lens pigments and macular xanthophyll pigment also absorb blue light, and phototoxic effects on the retina from blue light have been demonstrated. For these reasons, argon green is preferred over blue-green or blue alone.

The krypton laser delivers light energy of several wavelengths, and the red wavelength (647.1) has been used clinically. This red light is absorbed somewhat more deeply, producing burns within the RPE and choroid that expand to include the retina. Krypton laser has the advantage of passing through dispersed blood in the vitreous and through intraretinal hemorrhage more easily than does argon green and often is used to treat breaks in these settings. However, since the deeper uptake of this wavelength may cause Bruch's membrane rupture more frequently than argon green and since patients report more discomfort with krypton red treatment, argon green should be used unless significant vitreous or intraretinal hemorrhage prevents adequate laser uptake with the green wavelength.

The tunable dye laser produces a spectrum of continuously adjustable wavelengths and may be used to treat retinal breaks effectively. Since other laser wavelengths have not as yet demonstrated definite advantages over argon green and krypton red in the treatment of retinal breaks, discussion is limited to these two wavelengths.

Treatment Techniques

As previously mentioned, the goals of laser treatment are creation of a barrier around the break to prevent influx of vitreous fluid into the subretinal space and establishment of a firm adhesion around the tear to prevent further extension of the break. An understanding of the parameters of laser delivery will result in the proper application of laser and will accomplish these goals in a high percentage of cases.

Laser burn size, duration, power, and density are all important considerations for treatment and are summarized in Table 11–1. Most retinal breaks may be treated effectively with a 200 to 400 μm burn size using a standard Goldmann three-mirror or four-mirror contact lens with either argon or krypton laser. The use of the Rodenstock or Volk panfundus lens results in a larger burn area than indicated by the burn area setting on the laser. This effect necessitates a downward adjustment of the indicated burn size to produce burns consistent in size with the Goldmann-type lenses. Since shallow subretinal fluid may be more difficult to appreciate with the panfundus lenses because of peripheral distortion, mirrored lenses tend to be more effective for treatment of breaks associated with subclinical detachment.

TABLE 11–1. Treatment Parameters for Retinal Breaks

Spot Size	200–400 μm
Duration of Burn	0.1–0.2 sec
Initial Power Setting	150 mW
Wavelength	Argon green or krypton red
Contact Lens	Three- or four-mirror or panfundus
Anesthesia	Topical or retrobulbar

Goal: Medium-white laser burns spaced 100–200 μm apart in a honeycomb pattern. The entire lesion, including any subretinal fluid, should be enclosed by at least three rows of laser treatment.

*Increase laser power in 10–20 mW increments until appropriate burn appearance is attained.

*Adjust indicated burn size downward when using panfundus-type contact lens.

*Use krypton red with media opacity (i.e., vitreous hemorrhage, cataract) or intraretinal hemorrhage.

*To prevent Bruch's membrane rupture when using krypton, use 0.2-sec duration and begin at lower initial power setting. Consider retrobulbar anesthesia if patient discomfort limits effective treatment.

*Treat bridging retinal vessel concurrently if potential for vitreous hemorrhage appears significant.

The duration of laser burn should be 0.1 to 0.2 sec. Shorter burn durations require higher power levels to create an adequate chorioretinal adhesion of a given size. This combination may result in a greater incidence of Bruch's membrane rupture and intraretinal hemorrhage. Conversely, longer durations with lower power settings may result in fewer ruptures but are more painful and may interfere with adequate treatment due to increased patient discomfort. Although most patients can tolerate laser treatment with topical anesthetic only, extensive peripheral retinal pathologic conditions requiring a large amount of laser treatment may necessitate the use of a retrobulbar or peribulbar anesthetic. In these patients, the use of 0.1-sec burns allows for quick and efficient treatment. However, a laser duration of 0.2 sec with lower power settings is appropriate to minimize damage to Bruch's membrane.

Laser power is the most variable treatment parameter and is affected by the density of RPE pigmentation (light fundi require higher power; highly pigmented fundi require less power), the clarity of the ocular media (i.e., vitreous hemorrhage, cataract, posterior capsular opacity), and the presence of intraretinal hemorrhage or subretinal fluid. Determining the proper power for adequate treatment for a given eye is a matter of trial and error. The end point is a medium-white burn. Typically, using a 300 μm burn, the power level may be set initially at 150 mW for treatment of a peripheral tear using argon green through a three-mirror lens at 0.1-sec duration. Krypton laser requires a slightly lower initial setting because of deeper absorption and resultant increased tendency for Bruch's membrane rupture. Power is then increased in 10 to 20 mW increments until the desired burn appearance is attained. In gas-filled or silicone-filled eyes with clear media, power settings often are lower due to the insulating effects of the vitreous substitute.

The laser pattern should be uniform in appearance, and burns should be placed about 100 to 200 μm apart to prevent channels of subretinal fluid flowing between the burns within the treatment site. The most efficient burn distribution is a hexagonal or honeycomb laser pattern. Enough laser burns should be applied to surround the lesion with at least three rows of treatment (Fig. 11–3). The interface between attached retina and subretinal fluid should be visualized carefully so that the entire subclinical detachment is adequately contained within these three treatment rows. If intraretinal hemorrhage prevents laser uptake immediately adjacent to the lesion, laser burns should be extended beyond the hemorrhage to ensure successful treatment. Occasionally, an avulsed retinal vessel will be seen to bridge the gap between a flap tear and normal retina and may result in recurrent vitreous hemorrhage later. These bridging vessels can be treated effectively with argon green laser to produce vascular occlusion and to limit the potential for vitreous hemorrhage.[32]

Follow-up and Complications

After completion of laser therapy for symptomatic breaks, patients return for initial follow-up in 1 to 2 weeks. Patients with treated asymptomatic breaks may be seen in 2 to 4 weeks because of their decreased tendency to develop retinal detachment. More extensive breaks or those associated with subretinal fluid may need to be seen sooner because of potential instability. Superiorly oriented breaks also require earlier follow-up to rule out the possible accumulation of macula-threatening subretinal fluid. If the break demonstrates enlargement or if new subretinal fluid has appeared at the first examination, additional laser treatment should be administered at that time, with additional follow-up in 1 to 2 weeks.

The patient usually is scheduled for reexamination in 6 to 8 weeks if stable at the first follow-up appointment. Thereafter, yearly examinations should provide adequate follow-up for most patients.

Laser treatment applied in a careful fashion results in few complications. The most common is inadequate burn intensity, which produces an ineffective chorioretinal adhesion and places the patient at continued risk of detachment. As previously mentioned, ruptures in Bruch's membrane may occur if laser power is too high or burn size is too low. This tends not to cause difficulty,

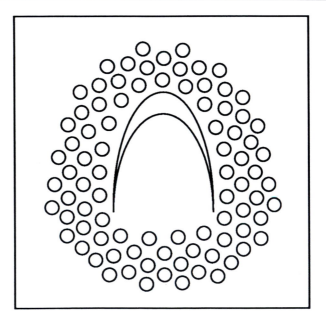

Figure 11–3. Honeycomb laser pattern for treatment of retinal breaks.

although an occasional patient will develop late choroidal neovascular activity at the rupture site. Intraretinal hemorrhage associated with excessive power may be visually significant if located close to the macula but usually resolves spontaneously. Vitreous hemorrhage from choroidal or retinal bleeding may render additional laser treatment more difficult but does not ordinarily decrease the visual prognosis. A full-thickness retinal hole may appear at a burn site if higher powers are used but is not typically associated with retinal detachment. Extensive laser treatment may stimulate epiretinal membrane formation, which can be visually threatening if the membrane extends to the perifoveal region. Such patients may require vitrectomy with membranectomy if sight is impaired significantly.

REFERENCES

1. Byer NE: Clinical study of retinal breaks. *Trans Am Acad Ophthalmol Otolaryngol* 1967;71:461–473.
2. Halpern JI: Routine screening of the retinal periphery. *Am J Ophthalmol* 1966;62: 99–102.
3. Rutnin U, Schepens CL: Fundus appearance in normal eyes: IV. Retinal breaks and other findings. *Am J Ophthalmol* 1967;64:1063–1078.
4. Neumann E, Hyams S: Conservative management of retinal breaks: a follow-up study of subsequent retinal detachment. *Br J Ophthalmol* 1972;56:482–486.
5. Balazs EA: Molecular morphology of the vitreous body. In: Smelser GK, ed. *The Structure of the Eye.* New York: Academic Press; 1961:293–310.
6. Hogan MJ, Alvarado JA, Weddell JE: *Histology of the Human Eye: An Atlas and Textbook.* Philadelphia: WB Saunders Co; 1971:611.
7. Sebag J: Age-related changes in human vitreous structure. *Graefe's Arch Clin Exp Ophthalmol* 1987;225:89–93.
8. Foos RY, Wheeler NC: Vitreoretinal juncture: synchysis senilis and posterior vitreous detachment. *Ophthalmology* 1982;89:1502–1512.
9. Hogan MJ: The vitreous, its structure, and relation to the ciliary body and retina. *Invest Ophthalmol* 1963;2:418–445.
10. Byer NE: Lattice degeneration of the retina. *Surv Ophthalmol* 1979;23:213–247.
11. Straatsma BR, Zeegen PD, Foos RY, Feman SS, Shabo AL: Lattice degeneration of the retina. *Trans Am Acad Ophthalmol Otolaryngol* 1974;78:87–113.
12. Byer NE: Changes in prognosis of lattice degeneration of the retina. *Trans Am Acad Ophthalmol Otolaryngol* 1974;78:114–125.
13. Ruben M, Rajpurohit P: Distribution of myopia in aphakic retinal detachments. *Br J Ophthalmol* 1976;60:517–521.
14. Folk JC, Burton TC: Bilateral phakic retinal detachment. *Ophthalmology* 1982;89: 815–820.
15. Rutnin U, Schepens CL: Fundus appearance in normal eyes: II. The standard peripheral fundus and developmental variations. *Am J Ophthalmol* 1967;64:840–852.
16. Tillery WV, Lucier AC: Round atrophic holes in lattice degeneration: an important cause of phakic retinal detachment. *Trans Am Acad Ophthalmol Otolaryngol* 1976; 81:509–518.
17. Scheie HG, Morse PH, Aminlari A: Incidence of retinal detachment following cataract extraction. *Arch Ophthalmol* 1973;89:293–295.
18. Coonan P, Fung WE, Webster RG Jr, Allen AW, Abbott RL: The incidence of retinal detachment following extracapsular cataract extraction: a ten-year study. *Ophthalmology* 1985;92:1096–1101.
19. Cox MS, Schepens CL, Freeman HM: Retinal detachment due to ocular contusion. *Arch Ophthalmol* 1966;76:678–685.
20. Sneed SR, Pulido JS, Blodi CF, Clarkson JG, Flynn HW Jr, Mieler WF: Surgical management of late-onset retinal detachments associated with regressed retinopathy of prematurity. *Ophthalmology* 1990;97:179–183.
21. Freeman WR, Henderly DE, Wan WL, Causey D, Trousdale M, Green RL, Rao NA: Prevalence, pathophysiology, and treatment of rhegmatogenous retinal detachment in treated *Cytomegalovirus* retinitis. *Am J Ophthalmol* 1987;103:527–536.

22. Blumenkranz MS, Culbertson WW, Clarkson JG, Dix R: Treatment of the acute retinal necrosis syndrome with intravenous acyclovir. *Ophthalmology* 1986;93: 296–300.
23. Nelson PT, Marcus DA, Bovino JA: Retinal detachment following endophthalmitis. *Ophthalmology* 1985;92:1112–1117.
24. Benson WE: *Retinal Detachment: Diagnosis and Management,* 2nd ed. Philadelphia: JB Lippincott; 1988:44–46.
25. Jaccoma EH, Conway BP, Campochiaro PA: Cryotherapy causes extensive breakdown of the blood–retinal barrier: a comparison with argon laser photocoagulation. *Arch Ophthalmol* 1985;103:1728–1730.
26. Campochiaro PA, Bryan JA III, Conway BP, Jaccoma EH: Intravitreal chemotactic and mitogenic activity: implication of blood–retinal barrier breakdown. *Arch Ophthalmol* 1986;104:1685–1687.
27. Campochiaro PA, Kaden IH, Vidaurri-Leal J, Glaser BM: Cryotherapy enhances intravitreal dispersion of viable retinal pigment epithelial cells. *Arch Ophthalmol* 1985; 103:434–436.
28. Zauberman H: Tensile strength of chorioretinal lesions produced by photocoagulation, diathermy, and cryopexy. *Br J Ophthalmol* 1969;53:749–752.
29. Lincoff H, O'Connor P, Bloch D, Nadel A, Kreissig I, Grinberg M: The cryosurgical adhesion: Part II. *Trans Am Acad Ophthalmol Otolaryngol* 1970;74:98–107.
30. Folk JC, Sneed SR, Folberg R, Coonan P, Pulido JS: Early retinal adhesion from laser photocoagulation. *Ophthalmology* 1989;96:1523–1525.
31. Yoon YH, Marmor MF: Recovery of retinal adhesivity, with and without photocoagulation, after experimental detachment in rabbits. *ARVO Abstract,* May 1–6, 1988.
32. Folk JC, Ma C, Blodi CF, Han DP: Occlusion of bridging or avulsed retinal vessels by repeated photocoagulation. *Ophthalmology* 1987;94:1610–1613.

CHAPTER 12

Laser Iridotomy

Wallace L. M. Alward

- ■ **Introduction**
- ■ **Indications**
- ■ **Laser Treatment**
  General Techniques
  Argon Laser Technique
  Neodymium:YAG Laser Technique
  Management After Iridotomy
  Complications
- ■ **References**

INTRODUCTION

Von Graefe introduced surgical iridectomy for glaucoma in 1857.[1] However, it was not until 1920 that Curran recognized that iridectomy was effective for angle-closure but not for open-angle glaucoma.[2] In 1956, Meyer-Schwickerath demonstrated that an iridotomy could be created without incision using xenon arc photocoagulation.[3] This failed to gain popularity because of frequent lens and corneal opacities. The pulsed ruby laser[4,5] and later the argon laser[6] were shown reliably to create iridotomies without the damage inflicted by the xenon arc system. Argon laser iridotomy and, more recently, neodymium:yttrium-aluminum-garnet (Nd:YAG) laser iridotomy have replaced surgical iridectomy as the primary treatment for angle-closure glaucoma.

Laser iridotomy has many advantages over surgical iridectomy. It causes little discomfort and, therefore, does not require retrobulbar or general anesthesia. The risks of intraocular surgery, such as wound leak, flat anterior chamber, cataract, infection, and serious hemorrhage, also are avoided. Surgical iridectomy is now used in eyes with severe inflammatory glaucoma with repeated closure of laser iridotomies, in eyes with opaque corneas, in those patients too ill or uncooperative to sit at the slit lamp, and when the laser is unavailable. Since the introduction of laser iridotomy, eyes with angle-closure glaucoma and their fellow eyes have been treated in a more timely fashion than in the surgical iridectomy era.[7]

INDICATIONS

The primary indication for laser peripheral iridotomy (LPI) is angle-closure glaucoma due to primary or secondary pupillary block. Secondary pupillary block can be caused by iris capture of an intraocular lens or by a secluded pupil from iridocyclitis. Acute, intermittent, and chronic pupillary block all are indications for laser peripheral iridotomy, as is the treatment of the fellow eye in a patient with angle-closure glaucoma in one eye. Laser peripheral iridotomy also aids in the diagnosis of plateau iris syndrome and malignant glaucoma. Neither condition can be diagnosed without the presence of a patent iridotomy or iridectomy. In patients with elevated intraocular pressure and narrow angles, laser iridotomy can establish whether the elevated pressure is primarily due to an open-angle or closed-angle process. The laser can be used to complete a partial-thickness surgical iridectomy. After an attack of malignant glaucoma in one eye, a prophylactic laser iridotomy in the fellow eye may avert a surgical iridectomy or a trabeculectomy, which would place the second eye at risk for the same problem. In nanophthalmic eyes, prophylactic iridotomies may preclude intraocular procedures that carry a high risk of suprachoroidal effusion.

Chronic angle closure due to neovascularization, inflammatory synechiae, or swelling of the ciliary body will not be helped by iridotomy, and it is important to recognize that the purpose of the laser iridotomy is to relieve pupillary block.

In eyes with cloudy corneas, widely dilated pupils, iridocorneal touch, or severe uveitis, it may not be possible to perform an iridotomy. If the eye has a severe anterior chamber reaction and a cloudy cornea, it often is best to control the intraocular pressure medically until the eye quiets. While waiting for the involved eye to become treatable, the clinician should consider an elective iridotomy in the uninvolved eye if there is symmetrical narrowing of the angles.

Both the argon and Nd:YAG lasers are safe and effective means of creating peripheral iridotomies.[8] The argon laser requires uptake of light energy by the pigment of the iris and is more difficult to use in lightly pigmented eyes. The photodisruptive Nd:YAG laser does not require pigmentation of the iris and works well on all iris colors. The Nd:YAG laser is somewhat quicker and requires less energy to create a patent iridotomy. It also has been reported to have fewer late closures than the argon laser.[8,9] In eyes with cloudy corneas, the Nd:YAG laser may be more effective in creating iridotomies than the argon laser. Because the Nd:YAG laser does not coagulate tissues, small hemorrhages occur in 35 to 45 percent of cases. These usually can be controlled easily with pressure on the contact lens.[8,9] The argon laser iridotomy can be crafted to have clean margins and is sometimes easier to evaluate for patency than is the often small, jagged iridotomy created by the Nd:YAG laser. For eyes with prominent vessels, the argon laser is preferable. A combination of the two lasers works well. The argon laser can be used to cut through the stroma, and a single low-power Nd:YAG application can clear away the pigment epithelium.

LASER TREATMENT

General Techniques

It is important to check the focus of the laser before beginning. Most lasers have a focusing bar that allows the surgeon to adjust the system to avoid the use of accommodation. The oculars are set on high plus, and each is slowly turned toward zero until a clear image is obtained. The magnification of the slit lamp should be rather high (about 25×) to give a shallow depth of field, which provides the most accurate focus. It is easiest to control laser delivery with the slit-lamp joystick than with the manipulator, which moves only the laser beam.

Corneal edema may preclude laser iridotomy during an acute attack of angle closure. The acute attack usually needs to be broken medically before iridotomy can be performed. The remaining corneal edema sometimes can be cleared with topical glycerine. In cases where the cornea is not clear enough for an iridotomy, the surgeon frequently can break an attack with argon laser iridoplasty or pupilloplasty.[10]

Miosis thins the iris and makes penetration easier. Pilocarpine should be delivered 1 hour before the iridotomy. Because apraclonidine can decrease the acute rise in pressure associated with iridotomies,[11] this should be given 1 hour before and immediately after the iridotomy. Topical anesthesia with an agent such as proparacaine is adequate for either argon or Nd:YAG iridotomy. Retrobulbar anesthesia is reserved for those few patients with severe nystagmus or difficulty with fixation.

For both lasers, the use of a contact lens makes the creation of an iridotomy easier and safer. The Abraham and Wise lenses are fitted with planoconvex buttons (66 D and 103 D, respectively) through which laser energy is focused. These lenses increase the cone angle and deliver more energy to the iris while delivering less energy to the cornea and retina. When compared to a plano contact lens, the energy delivered to the iris is increased 2.67-fold for the Abraham lens and 7.79-fold for the Wise lens.[12] The energy delivered to the cornea is decreased to 36 percent with the Abraham lens and 9 percent with the Wise lens when compared to a plano lens.[12] Similarly, the retinal energy is decreased to 37 percent with the Abraham lens and 9 percent with the Wise lens.[12] The contact lens also serves to keep the lids open and helps to decrease eye movements. The lens and the methylcellulose act as a heat sink. The lens should have an antireflective coating to increase the delivery of energy to the iris.

The iridotomy should be placed in the midperipheral iris (Fig. 12–1). It should be peripheral enough to clear areas of iris–lens touch but not be so peripheral that it is difficult to evaluate under an arcus senilis. If placed in the hazy peripheral cornea, there is an increased chance of corneal burns, a decreased uptake by the iris, and more difficulty in determining the patency of the iridotomy once the miotic has worn off. The iridotomies should be placed under the upper eyelid to avoid extra images through a second pupil. The 12:00

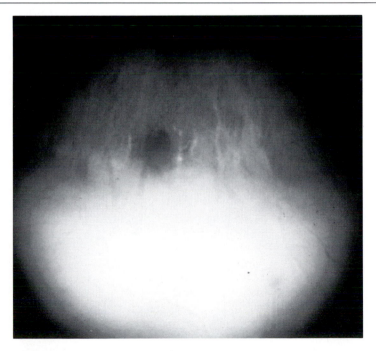

Figure 12–1. Argon laser peripheral iridotomy in the superior peripheral iris.

o'clock position is avoided because bubbles can accumulate and impair the completion of the iridotomy. The superonasal location has the theoretical advantage of decreasing the risk to the macula. Regardless of location, the beam should be angled away from the macula. If iris crypts are present, they represent relatively thin areas that may make penetration easier. In light irides, one can place an argon laser iridotomy at a freckle to increase the chance of penetration. When the iris seems to be particularly difficult to penetrate in one location, it is sometimes helpful to try another site. A cloud of pigment and deepening of the anterior chamber suggest penetration. However, seeing the lens capsule or zonules through the iridotomy is the only way to be sure of patency. In some aphakic eyes, the adherence of vitreous over the posterior iris can necessitate more than one iridotomy to find access to the aqueous.

With capture of an intraocular lens, there is sometimes dramatic iris bombe around the lens, which places the iris dangerously close to the corneal endothelium. In this instance, it is best to make an iridotomy next to the lens optic or haptic where the chamber is held deeper by the intraocular lens. Once the chamber deepens, a midperipheral iridotomy can be created safely. The original iridotomy often will slide under the intraocular lens once the pupil constricts and cannot be relied on for preventing further attacks.

Argon Laser Technique

There are many techniques for creating an iridotomy with the continuous wave argon laser. These techniques can be modified based on iris color and individual iris reaction.

The direct technique employs a 50 μm spot that is applied with a power of about 1 W for 0.02 to 0.2 sec (Table 12–1). Shorter duration burns typically are used on darker irides, which char with long burns.[13] Short duration burns delivered through the Wise lens can cause evaporation of tissue without char.[12] Longer duration burns (0.2 sec and longer) are sometimes helpful for light-colored irides[14] but may be more uncomfortable. Longer duration burns may provide better hemostasis in eyes with neovascularization. A single area is treated with continued applications of energy until perforation is obtained. Frequently, gas bubbles will form.

TABLE 12–1. Argon Laser Peripheral Iridotomy

Spot Size	50 μm
Duration	0.02–0.2 sec
Initial Power	1000 mW
Wavelength	Argon blue-green
Contact Lens	Abraham or Wise
Anesthesia	Topical

Goal: To create an opening through the iris that will enable aqueous to pass freely from the posterior chamber to the anterior chamber.

Note: Pretreat with pilocarpine and apraclonidine. The iridotomy should be placed in the peripheral iris beneath the upper lid to prevent the patient from seeing extra images. Direct the beam away from the macula. Adjust the power and duration based on iris color (see text). For very light or thick irides, consider the Nd:YAG laser. Give apraclonidine immediately after the treatment. Place the patient on a short course of topical corticosteroids postoperatively.

These will float away or will move with the next application. A patent iridotomy usually can be created during one session, although some difficult eyes may require more than one session.

If the pigment epithelial layer is difficult to clear away, lower power settings may prevent the sliding of pigment into the iridotomy.[15] Alternatively, a single low energy spot with the Nd:YAG laser can remove the remaining pigment readily. This must be done with caution to prevent lens capsule damage, and initial Nd:YAG energy of 1 mJ or less should be used.

If penetration is difficult with the argon laser, one can switch to the Nd:YAG laser. The Nd:YAG laser has been shown to be effective in cases where the argon laser has failed.[16]

For those surgeons without access to a Nd:YAG laser, there are several alternate techniques described for penetration of the iris with argon energy. Abraham and Miller have described a technique in which a single preparatory spot (100–500 μm, 500 mW, 0.2–0.5 sec) is placed in the 3:00 or 9:00 o'clock position, which causes the iris to hump, leaving thin iris above and below. Penetrating burns (50–200 μm, 500–1800 mW, 0.2–1.0 sec) are placed in the thinned iris on the superior hump.[17] Another technique has been described in which four preparatory spots (50 μm, 200–300 mW, 0.2–0.5 sec) put an area of iris on stretch, and penetration is carried out in the taut area with shorter, more intense burns (50 μm, 500–2000 mW, 0.1–0.2 sec).[18] Other techniques of stretching and penetrating have been described.[19,20] The radial tension in the iris can be used to pull open a large iridotomy. In this technique, a linear cut is made across the iris fibers (50 μm, 800–1500 mW, 0.02 sec, Abraham or CGI lens), and the inherent iris tension opens an iridotomy.[21]

Neodymium:YAG Laser Technique

Unlike the thermal effects of the argon laser, the Q-switched Nd:YAG laser uses photodisruption and does not require iris pigmentation to be effective (Table 12–2). In one large study it successfully created an iridotomy in 99 percent of 200 eyes.[22] Because the Nd:YAG light is invisible, a helium-neon aiming beam is used to direct the laser energy. The aiming beam is brought to a focus by joining two or more beams into a single spot.

TABLE 12–2. Neodymium:YAG Laser Peripheral Iridotomy

Spot Size	Fixed
Duration	Fixed nanoseconds
Initial Energy	1–12 mJ
Wavelength	Nd:YAG
Contact Lens	Abraham, Wise, or Lasag CGI
Anesthesia	Topical

Goal: To create an opening through the iris that will enable aqueous to pass freely from the posterior chamber to the anterior chamber.

Note: Pretreat with pilocarpine and apraclonidine. The iridotomy should be placed in the peripheral iris beneath the upper lid to prevent the patient from seeing extra images. Direct the beam away from the macula. When enlarging an iridotomy, direct the laser energy to strands of iris at the side of the opening. Avoid firing onto the lens capsule. Control any bleeding with pressure on the contact lens. Give apraclonidine immediately after the treatment. Place the patient on a short course of topical corticosteroids postoperatively.

The same locations are used as for an argon iridotomy—in the midperipheral iris, usually superonasally, and in a crypt if one is available (Fig. 12–2). The possibility of disrupting the lens capsule is higher with the Nd:YAG laser, and it is, therefore, more important to be peripheral than with the argon laser. The laser aiming beam is focused on the anterior iris stroma, and the energy is delivered in single bursts or in chains of 2 to 3 bursts. With the Abraham lens, an energy setting of 3 to 5 mJ is used (higher energy levels have been described but are not usually necessary). With the Wise lens, energy settings as low as 1 mJ can be employed.[12] When the laser cone angle is adjustable, it is best to choose a high cone angle and minimize risk to the cornea and retina. Some lasers give the option of fundamental mode and multimode operation. The fundamental mode uses only the energy in the center of the cone and may be useful in tight places. The multimode requires a lower energy setting than the fundamental mode and typically is preferred.

The iridotomy usually is created with 1 to 10 applications. If the iris is difficult to penetrate, the surgeon can increase the energy carefully or try a different site. If the view is impaired by blood, pigment, or corneal changes, it may be necessary to complete the iridotomy on another day.

When enlarging an iridotomy, it is necessary to avoid applications directly over the lens capsule. Additional spots are best delivered to adjacent iris.

Management After Iridotomy

Immediately after iridotomy, a second drop of apraclonidine is administered. The intraocular pressure is checked 1 or 2 hours later. If the pressure is adequate, the patient is discharged on topical prednisolone four times daily for 4 days. Preoperative glaucoma medications are continued. Some surgeons prefer to have patients continue to take pilocarpine for several weeks because of the possibility of closure of the iridotomy.[15] Others prefer to dilate immediately after iridotomy.[23]

On follow-up examination, the iridotomy is inspected for patency. The lens capsule should be visible through the iridotomy in phakic patients.

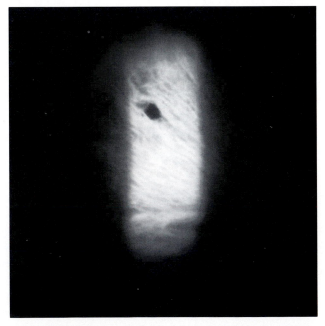

Figure 12–2. YAG peripheral iridotomy in the superior mid peripheral iris.

Despite a red reflex through the iridotomy, there may be a translucent membrane remaining. Gonioscopy is repeated to evaluate the degree to which the angle has opened, to identify areas of synechial closure, and to determine whether the patient has an element of plateau iris syndrome. The eye is then dilated to evaluate the optic nerve and retina. If the patient has had angle closure in one eye, the other eye deserves careful evaluation and usually will require a prophylactic iridotomy unless there is a marked asymmetry between the eyes.

Complications

After iridotomy, patients frequently note blurred vision due to pigment release and sometimes due to hemorrhage. This clears spontaneously.

All eyes treated with either laser will have a transient iritis,[24] and, therefore, patients are placed on a short course of corticosteroids. The Nd:YAG laser may cause somewhat less inflammation than the argon laser.[9,24] Occasionally, inflammation can be quite severe, and posterior synechiae may develop.[17] When evaluating an eye shortly after an iridotomy, there will be abundant pigment in the anterior chamber, which should not be mistaken for cells.

There is a transient elevation of intraocular pressure in about one third of eyes treated with either laser.[18,24] The pressure rise can be quite dramatic,[25] and it is important to check the intraocular pressure 1 to 2 hours after iridotomy. The use of apraclonidine has been shown to decrease the risk of intraocular pressure elevation significantly. In a masked study of apraclonidine vs placebo, intraocular pressure spikes of 10 mm Hg or more occurred in 43 percent of the placebo eyes and in none of the apraclonidine-treated eyes after iridotomy.[11]

Corneal epithelial opacities can develop, especially if the beam is poorly focused or the power setting is especially high. In very shallow anterior chambers, there can be corneal endothelial opacities because energy is delivered so close to the cornea.[26] In a long-term follow-up of argon laser iridotomies, no evidence of clinically significant corneal endothelial damage was found in normal corneas.[27] However, in eyes with marginally compensated corneas, there have been cases of corneal decompensation.[28] After Nd:YAG laser iridotomy, Descemet's membrane and corneal stroma can appear to be shattered.[8] Although visible corneal changes usually are transient, irreversible endothelial cell loss has been demonstrated with Nd:YAG laser iridotomy.[29] The use of a magnifying contact lens (Abraham, Wise, CGI) decreases the amount of laser energy delivered to the cornea and offers considerable protection from damage.[12]

Punctate lens epithelial changes can be seen after argon and Nd:YAG laser iridotomy.[17,18,24] These changes do not progress to cataract. With the Nd:YAG laser, there is more potential for serious lens damage. Anterior capsular and zonular rupture have been reported with the Nd:YAG laser.[30,31]

Bleeding occurs frequently with Nd:YAG iridotomies but rarely with argon iridotomies. One study found that 44 percent of eyes bled after Nd:YAG treatment vs no bleeding after argon treatment.[8] Bleeding is stopped usually by applying pressure to the eye with the contact lens.

Retinal damage, including foveal damage with visual loss, can occur with laser iridotomy.[32] Risk to the retina can be minimized by using a contact lens, by avoiding high energy levels, and by directing the beam away from the fovea.

Closure of the iridotomy can occur. This is more likely if the iridotomy is small or if the eye has anterior chamber inflammation. Closure of an argon laser iridotomy is more common than is closure of a Nd:YAG laser iridotomy.[8,9,22] When closure occurs, it is usually within the first few weeks.[8]

Monocular diplopia can occur if the iridotomy is not covered by the lid. Therefore, iridotomies in the palpebral fissure should be avoided when possible.[26]

The pupil may peak toward an argon laser iridotomy[17] (especially with long burns) and occasionally toward a Nd:YAG laser iridotomy.[22] Pilocarpine may protect against pupil distortion. When the pupil does peak, it usually returns to a normal shape.[23]

REFERENCES

1. Von Graefe A: Über die Iridectomie bei Glaucom und über den glaucomatosen Process. *Graefes Arch Clin Exp Ophthalmol* 1857;3(pt 2):456–555.
2. Curran EJ: A new operation for glaucoma involving a new principle in the etiology and treatment of chronic primary glaucoma. *Arch Ophthalmol* 1920;49:131–155.
3. Meyer-Schwickerath G: Erfahrungen mit der Lichtkoagulation der Netzhaut und der Iris. *Doc Ophthalmol* 1956;10:91–131.
4. Snyder WB: Laser coagulation of the anterior segment: I. Experimental laser iridotomy. *Arch Ophthalmol* 1967;77:93–98.
5. Perkins ES: Laser iridotomy. *Br Med J* 1970;2:580–581.
6. Khuri CH: Argon laser iridectomies. *Am J Ophthalmol* 1973;76:490–493.
7. Rivera AH, Brown RH, Anderson DR: Laser iridotomy vs surgical iridectomy: have the indications changed? *Arch Ophthalmol* 1985;103:1350–1354.
8. Del Priore LV, Robin AL, Pollack IP: Neodymium:YAG and argon laser iridotomy: long-term follow-up in a prospective, randomized clinical trial. *Ophthalmology* 1988; 95:1207–1211.
9. Moster MR, Schwartz LW, Spaeth GL, Wilson RP, McAllister JA, Poryzees EM: Laser iridectomy: a controlled study comparing argon and neodymium:YAG. *Ophthalmology* 1986;93:20–24.
10. Ritch R: Argon laser treatment for medically unresponsive attacks of angle-closure. *Am J Ophthalmol* 1982;94:197–204.
11. Robin AL, Pollack IP, deFaller JM: Effects of topical ALO 2145 (*p*-aminoclonidine hydrochloride) on the acute intraocular pressure rise after argon laser iridotomy. *Arch Ophthalmol* 1987;105:1208–1211.
12. Wise JB, Munnerlyn CR, Erickson PJ: A high-efficiency laser iridotomy-sphincterotomy lens. *Am J Ophthalmol* 1986;101:546–553.
13. Ritch R, Palmberg P: Argon laser iridectomy in densely pigmented irides. *Am J Ophthalmol* 1982;93:800–801.
14. Hoskins HD, Migliazzo CV: Laser iridectomy—a technique for blue irises. *Ophthalmic Surg* 1984;15:488–490.
15. Shields MB: *Textbook of Glaucoma*, 2nd ed. Baltimore: Williams & Wilkins; 1987:450.
16. Robin AL, Pollack IP: Q-switched neodymium-YAG laser iridotomy in patients in whom the argon laser fails. *Arch Ophthalmol* 1986;104:531–535.
17. Abraham RK, Miller GL: Outpatient argon laser iridectomy for angle-closure glaucoma: A two-year study. *Trans Am Acad Ophthalmol Otolaryngol* 1975;79:529–538.
18. Pollack IP, Patz A: Argon laser iridotomy: an experimental and clinical study. *Ophthalmic Surg* 1976;7:22–30.
19. Mandelkorn RM, Mendelsohn AD, Olander KW, Zimmerman TJ: Short exposure times in argon laser iridotomy. *Ophthalmic Surg* 1981;12:805–809.
20. Podos SM, Kels BD, Moss AP, Ritch R, Anders MD: Continuous wave argon laser iridectomy in angle-closure glaucoma. *Am J Ophthalmol* 1979;88:836–842.
21. Wise JB: Iris sphincterotomy, iridotomy, and synechiotomy by linear incision with the argon laser. *Ophthalmology* 1985;92:641–645.
22. Schwartz LW, Moster MR, Spaeth GL, Wilson RP, Poryzees E: Neodymium-YAG laser iridectomies in glaucoma associated with closed or occludable angles. *Am J Ophthalmol* 1986;102:41–44.
23. Abraham RK: Protocol for single-session argon laser iridectomy for angle-closure glaucoma. *Int Ophthalmol Clin* 1981;21:145–166.
24. Robin AL, Pollack IP: A comparison of neodymium:YAG and argon laser iridotomies. *Ophthalmology* 1984;91:1011–1016.

25. Krupin T, Stone RA, Cohen BH, Kolker AE, Kass MA: Acute intraocular pressure response to argon laser iridotomy. *Ophthalmology* 1985;92:922–926.
26. Pollack IP: Use of argon laser energy to produce iridotomies. *Trans Am Ophthalmol Soc* 1979;77:674–706.
27. Thoming C, Van Buskirk EM, Samples JR: The corneal endothelium after laser therapy for glaucoma. *Am J Ophthalmol* 1987;103:518–522.
28. Schwartz AL, Martin NF, Weber PA: Corneal decompensation after argon laser iridectomy. *Arch Ophthalmol* 1988;106:1572–1574.
29. Kerr Muir MG, Sherrard ES: Damage to the corneal endothelium during Nd/YAG photodisruption. *Br J Ophthalmol* 1985;69:77–85.
30. Berger CM, Lee DA, Christensen RE: Anterior lens perforation and zonular rupture after Nd:YAG laser iridotomy. *Am J Ophthalmol* 1989;107:674–675.
31. Welch DB, Apple DJ, Mendelsohn AD, Reidy JJ, Chalkley THF, Wilensky JT: Lens injury following iridotomy with a Q-switched neodymium-YAG laser. *Arch Ophthalmol* 1986;104:123–125.
32. Berger BB: Foveal photocoagulation from laser iridotomy. *Ophthalmology* 1984;91: 1029–1033.

CHAPTER 13

Argon Laser Trabeculoplasty

Wallace L.M. Alward

- ■ Introduction
- ■ Indications
- ■ Mechanism
- ■ Laser Treatment
  Technique
  Complications
  Retreatment
- ■ References

INTRODUCTION

Early laser treatments for open-angle glaucoma were attempts to puncture through the trabecular meshwork and into Schlemm's canal.[1-3] The lowered pressure from these procedures was generally short-lived. In the early 1970s, extensive nonpenetrating laser treatment of the trabecular meshwork was used to create experimental glaucoma in monkeys.[4] In 1979, Wise and Witter demonstrated that small, nonpenetrating laser burns scattered around the angle could lower intraocular pressure in humans and that the results were long-lasting.[5] Argon laser trabeculoplasty has gained widespread acceptance and has replaced trabeculectomy as the first surgical procedure on eyes with open-angle glaucoma. Trabeculoplasty decreases the intraocular pressure in over 80 percent of eyes with primary open-angle glaucoma.[5,6] The drop in intraocular pressure usually is in the range of 7 to 13 mm Hg[5,7,8] and is proportional to the preoperative intraocular pressure.[6]

INDICATIONS

Laser trabeculoplasty is used to control elevated intraocular pressure in those patients with open-angle glaucoma in whom medical therapy has failed to bring about control. It is effective in primary open-angle glaucoma and in some secondary open-angle glaucomas, such as pseudoexfoliative and pigmentary glaucoma.[6] Some pressure lowering has been demonstrated in low-tension glaucoma, especially in those with intraocular pressures at the higher end of the normal range.[6,9] It also can be used successfully after failed filtering operations.[6] Trabeculoplasty is less effective in aphakia, congenital glaucoma, angle recession glaucoma, and inflammatory glaucoma.[5,6,8] It works best in those over 40 years of age,[6] and although equally effective in blacks and whites,[10] the pressure-lowering effect does not appear to be as long-lasting in blacks.[11] Laser trabeculoplasty is, of course, not indicated and not possible in primary angle-closure glaucoma. It also is of little use to treat an eye with chronic angle-closure in which more than 180 degrees of the mesh-work is permanently closed by synechiae.

Eyes with symmetrical disease tend to respond similarly to trabeculo-plasty.[12]

MECHANISM

In laser trabeculoplasty, tiny, nonpenetrating burns are placed in the trabecu-lar meshwork for 180 to 360 degrees of the circumference. The mechanism by which these burns cause an increased aqueous outflow[7] and a decreased intraocular pressure is not clear. At the site of laser energy absorption, there is thinning and scarring and no evidence of flow.[13] Laser trabeculoplasty increases outflow between the laser burns where the spaces between the tra-becular beams are widened and free of debris.[13] Wise and Witter proposed a mechanical tightening of the trabecular ring to account for the increase in out-flow.[5,14] With the loss of treated endothelial cells, the remaining trabecular cells demonstrate an increase in cell division[15] and phagocytosis.[16] This increase in biologic activity and alteration of the extracellular matrix[17] may improve trabecular function.

LASER TREATMENT

Technique

Because intraocular pressure elevation is common after laser trabeculoplasty, apraclonidine is administered 1 hour before treatment and immediately after-ward to avert or decrease any intraocular pressure elevation.

Accurate placement of the laser energy is critical for this procedure, and the surgeon should assure adequate focus of the slit lamp before proceeding. The slit-lamp oculars are fogged with high plus and are then individually focused on the aiming bar to provide clear focus without accommodation. A slit-lamp magnification of 16× to 25× works well. The patient's lateral can-thus should be aligned with the canthal mark on the slit lamp to allow ade-quate excursion of the laser delivery system during treatment. For many surgeons, an elbow rest is useful to assist in holding the goniolens steadily and comfortably.

Treatment usually is administered through the smallest (59 degrees) mir-ror of a Goldmann three-mirror lens with antireflective coating. A Goldmann one-mirror lens can be used in patients with tight lid fissures. An alternative to the Goldmann lenses is the Ritch lens, which has four mirrors directed into the angle, two of which have magnifying lenses to focus the beam more tightly.

A spot size of 50 μm is selected with a duration of 0.1 sec. Treatment usu-ally is initiated with a power setting of 600 to 700 mW. If the angle is heavily pigmented, the surgeon should begin at a lower power. The aiming beam is kept dim to protect the surgeon from excessive light exposure and to allow the most critical focusing. If there are annoying reflections, the illuminating por-tion of the slit lamp can be decentered slightly (Table 13–1).

TABLE 13–1. Argon Laser Trabeculoplasty

Spot Size	50 μm
Duration	0.1 sec
Power Setting	200–1200 mW
Wavelength	Argon blue-green
Contact Lens	Goldmann three-mirror
Anesthesia	Topical

Goal: To treat 180 degrees of the trabecular meshwork with argon laser energy in order to increase the facility of aqueous outflow.

Note: One hour before treatment, the eye is given 1 drop of apraclonidine. The Goldmann three-mirror lens is coupled to the anesthetized eye with methylcellulose. The laser energy is delivered through the short mirror of the three-mirror lens. The beam is aimed at the junction of the pigmented and nonpigmented trabecular meshwork. The laser power is adjusted to cause blanching of the trabecular tissues or slight bubble formation. One should avoid excessive tissue reaction. Applications are placed 2 or 3 beam widths apart. Forty to fifty applications are delivered per 180 degrees. On completion, a drop of apraclonidine is instilled in the eye. The patient is placed on a short course of topical corticosteroids.

Topical anesthesia with 0.5 percent proparacaine usually is adequate. Retrobulbar anesthesia is rarely needed in patients with nystagmus or poor fixation.

The inferior 180 degrees normally is treated first. The inferior angle is usually the widest and the most pigmented and has the clearest landmarks. It is important to have a routine so that if the patient returns for a second treatment, it is known what was done during the first session, even if the records cannot be located. The Goldmann lens is filled with methylcellulose and applied to the anesthetized eye with the short mirror in the 9 o'clock position. The slit lamp is focused on the trabecular meshwork 180 degrees away from the mirror (the 3 o'clock trabecular meshwork), and the aiming beam is positioned over the junction of the pigmented and nonpigmented trabecular meshwork. The beam should strike perpendicular to the meshwork so that it can be sharply focused. The physician may need to tilt the lens or ask the patient to redirect his or her gaze to achieve crisp focus. If the beam is not perpendicular, it becomes oblong and decreases the energy delivered. The position of the laser beam is best adjusted with the slit-lamp joystick rather than the laser manipulator. Proper placement of the burns is important (Fig. 13–1). If the burns are placed posteriorly, there is more chance of developing inflammation and synechiae.[18] Applications on the cornea have been associated with overgrowth of endothelium over the meshwork.[19] A clear understanding of the gonioscopic landmarks is essential for performing laser trabeculoplasty. If the surgeon is having difficulty separating landmarks in the angle, a thin slit beam obliquely illuminated into the angle should demonstrate two corneal lines forming a corneal wedge. The outer line represents the corneal epithelium, and the inner line represents the corneal endothelium. These lines join at Schwalbe's line, which marks the anterior border of the trabecular meshwork. This technique is especially valuable in lightly pigmented angles.

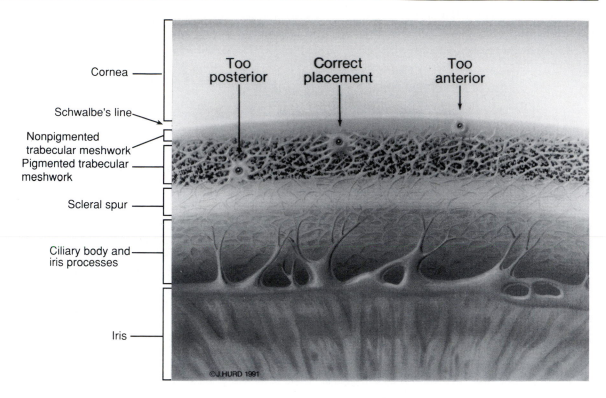

Cornea

Schwalbe's line

Nonpigmented trabecular meshwork

Pigmented trabecular meshwork

Scleral spur

Ciliary body and iris processes

Iris

Too posterior

Correct placement

Too anterior

©J.HURD 1991

Figure 13–1. Diagram of anterior chamber angle, demonstrating the range of treatment response to argon laser treatment. *(Reprinted courtesy of Schwartz A, Hurd J.)*

After the initial laser burns, the power is adjusted to give a minimal tissue reaction, blanching or a small bubble (Fig. 13–2). If there are large bubbles or a shower of pigment, the energy level needs to be decreased. The use of excessive power has been associated with more synechiae.[18] If the meshwork is nonpigmented, the tissue reaction may not be visible. In this situation, a maximal power of 1000 to 1200 mW should be employed. A therapeutic effect probably will occur despite the lack of apparent uptake. The inferior 180 degrees is treated with 40 to 50 applications, and at a second sitting, the remaining 180 degrees may be treated.

The most difficult aspect of laser trabeculoplasty is maintaining orientation as the mirror is moved from site to site. Because the energy is delivered through a mirror, it is difficult to administer a row of burns and then turn the mirror and find where the therapy should be resumed. If the angle is pigmented and blanches well, it is relatively easy to find where one has left off, but in lightly pigmented angles, it is easy to become lost. The surgeon may find it easiest to begin at 3 o'clock (mirror at 9 o'clock) and to turn the lens clockwise slightly after every few burns, always using the center portion of the mirror. This constant turning of the lens avoids having to make large turns where orientation could be lost. If large turns of the lens are required, it is important to pick landmarks, such as freckles or iris crypts, as reference points to allow accurate placement of the next burn. Treatment is continued until the 9 o'clock angle (mirror in the 3 o'clock position) is reached.

Narrow angles are more difficult to treat. If there is a large degree of pupillary block, a peripheral iridotomy may be necessary before trabeculoplasty. Usually, the approach to the angle is only somewhat steep, and having the patient look in the direction of the mirror will improve access to the meshwork. In some patients, argon laser iridoplasty is required to flatten the

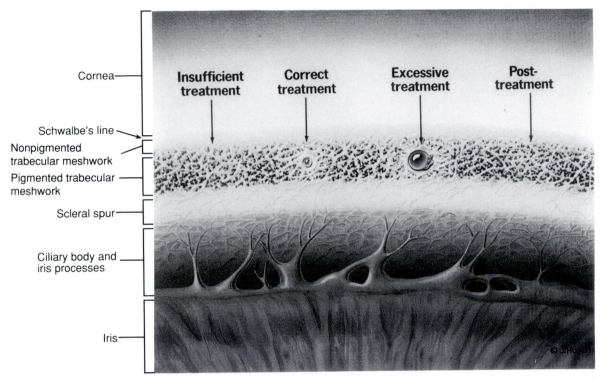

Figure 13–2. Diagram of anterior chamber angle, demonstrating the correct placement of laser treatment to the junction of the pigmented and non pigmented trabecular meshwork. *(Reprinted courtesy of Schwartz A, Hurd J, from* Ophthalmology *1981;88:pp. 203–212.)*

iris in front of the angle and provide an adequate view. This is accomplished by applying large, long, low-powered burns to the far peripheral iris, either through the goniolens or without a lens.

Laser iridoplasty (Table 13–2) usually is performed using 500 μm spots at 0.5 sec and 150 to 300 mW, delivered to the far peripheral iris without a lens, watching for visible shrinkage of tissue (Fig. 13–3).

TABLE 13–2. Argon Laser Iridoplasty

Spot Size	200–500 μm
Duration	0.2–0.5 sec
Power Setting	150–300 mW
Wavelength	Argon blue-green
Contact Lens	None or Goldmann
Anesthesia	Topical

Goal: To shrink iris tissue and pull it from the angle.

Note: Pilocarpine puts the iris on stretch. The laser is aimed at the far peripheral iris, just inside the limbus. A long, low-power laser application should cause visible contraction of iris tissue without charring. Applications are spaced regularly over 360 degrees of the iris surface (usually 4–6 applications per quadrant). The patient is placed on a short course of topical corticosteroids.

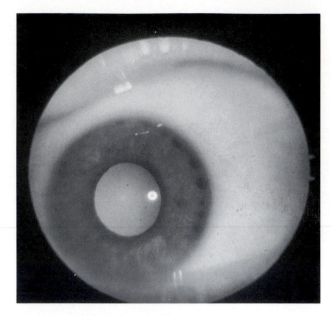

Figure 13–3. Laser iridoplasty to the far peripheral iris using a large spot size.

If the angle has peripheral anterior synechiae, it is probably best to avoid laser trabeculoplasty of the open angle immediately adjacent to the synechiae because inflammation may cause the synechiae to spread.

Immediately after laser trabeculoplasty, a second drop of apraclonidine is administered, and the intraocular pressure is checked over the next 1 to 2 hours. If the pressure rises, the patient is treated with beta-blockers, cholinergics, carbonic anhydrase inhibitors, and osmotic agents as needed to control the pressure. Often, osmotics are the only agents the patient is not already taking. The patient is monitored until the pressure has come down and stayed down after the osmotic agent has worn off. Patients with very high pressure or extremely damaged nerves may need to be observed up to 6 hours to detect late pressure elevations.[20]

Topical corticosteroids are administered four times daily for 4 days in addition to any preexisting glaucoma medications. The results of the trabeculoplasty may not be stable for weeks. Patients are seen about 6 weeks after completion of the trabeculoplasty to determine whether the treatment has been effective. If there has been a dramatic reduction in intraocular pressure, one can cautiously begin reducing some glaucoma medications. As a general rule, however, most patients need to keep using their pretreatment medications.

In addition to intraocular pressure measurement, the posttreatment evaluation should include slit-lamp biomicroscopy to look for signs of iritis and gonioscopy to look for evidence of synechiae formation.

Complications

In comparison with filtering surgery, complications of laser trabeculoplasty are uncommon and, for the most part, mild.

The most common serious sequela to laser trabeculoplasty is a rise in intraocular pressure.[6,20,21] This occurs almost immediately and occasionally is marked enough to place the optic nerve in jeopardy, as evidenced by the loss of visual field[20,21] and central vision.[6] In one study, 3 percent of eyes had a permanent increase in intraocular pressure.[6] The cause of the pressure rise is unknown. Histopathologic studies have demonstrated an accumulation of inflammatory cells and debris within the meshwork.[22] Animal studies have suggested that the release of prostaglandin-like substances may contribute to a decrease in outflow and an increase in intraocular pressure.[23]

One way to avoid large intraocular pressure spikes is to treat no more than 180 degrees of the angle at a time; 360 degrees therapy has been shown to have a greater tendency to elevate the intraocular pressure[6,24] and does not lower the intraocular pressure more than does 180 degrees of therapy.[24] Pilocarpine can prevent some of the pressure rise,[25] but most patients who come to trabeculoplasty are already taking pilocarpine. Apraclonidine has been shown to be effective at limiting intraocular pressure spikes after trabeculoplasty. One study found a postoperative pressure spike in 59 percent of the placebo group and in 21 percent of the apraclonidine-treated group. Spikes in pressure over 10 mm Hg were seen in 18 percent of the placebo group and none of the apraclonidine group.[26]

Small white corneal opacities can develop during treatment. These are never large enough to interrupt the treatment and generally clear in a few days. Trabeculoplasty does not appear to cause permanent corneal endothelial damage.[27]

Iritis may follow trabeculoplasty[7] but usually is suppressed by the corticosteroids administered after the treatment. Trabeculitis may produce white keratic precipitates on the trabecular meshwork and cause the intraocular pressure to go up during the first few weeks after treatment. The precipitates will resolve and the intraocular pressure will go down with intensive topical corticosteroid treatment. Peripheral anterior synechiae occur commonly if the posterior part of the meshwork is treated.[6] If the energy is delivered to the middle of the meshwork, synechiae are uncommon.

Hemorrhage can occur on occasion and usually is stopped easily by applying pressure to the contact lens[6] or by applying low-power 200 micron burns to the bleeding area.[14]

Syncope is infrequent.[21] Cystoid macular edema occurs rarely in aphakic eyes.[21]

Treatment failures occur in about 20 percent of eyes and are seen more often in young patients, in aphakic patients, in congenital glaucoma, in inflammatory glaucoma, in angle recession glaucoma, and in some other secondary glaucomas. After an adequate response, there is a gradual loss of control at a rate of 7 to 10 percent per year over the first 5 years.[28,29] Most delayed failures seem to occur in the first year.[29] If a patient has had inadequate response to trabeculoplasty in one eye, the physician should not be optimistic about achieving a good response in the fellow eye.[12]

Retreatment

If the patient has had 180 degrees of treatment, completing the therapy at a later date is reasonable. If the patient has undergone 360 degrees of trabeculoplasty in one or more sessions and years later has an elevation of intraocular pressure, retreatment is controversial. Studies have shown a decrease in intraocular pressure in 36 to 73 percent of patients after repeat trabeculoplasty.[30–33] The major concern with repeat trabeculoplasty is the tendency for marked pressure elevation.[30–32] Brown and co-workers found that 10 (38 percent) of 26 eyes that had initial success with laser trabeculoplasty demonstrated an elevation of intraocular pressure after repeat treatment. The intraocular pressure in these eyes rose by as much as 37 mm Hg, and 8 of the 10 eyes with an elevated pressure required filtering surgery within 1 month because of progressive optic nerve or visual field changes.[31] Messner and associates had similar results, with 50 percent of those undergoing repeat trabeculoplasty requiring filtering surgery within 6 months.[32] Conversely, Jorizzo and co-workers found no significant rise in intraocular pressure among 11 retreated patients.[33]

Repeat trabeculoplasty should be restricted to patients who had an initial satisfactory and prolonged response to trabeculoplasty. The patient should be warned of the substantial risk for pressure elevation, which may require urgent surgical treatment.

REFERENCES

1. Worthen DM, Wickham MG: Argon laser trabeculotomy. *Trans Am Acad Ophthalmol Otolaryngol* 1974;78:371–375.
2. Ticho U, Zauberman H: Argon laser application to the angle structures in the glaucomas. *Arch Ophthalmol* 1976;94:61–64.
3. Krasnov MM: Laseropuncture of anterior chamber angle in glaucoma. *Am J Ophthalmol* 1973;75:674–678.
4. Gaasterland D, Kupfer C: Experimental glaucoma in the rhesus monkey. *Invest Ophthalmol* 1974;13:455–457.
5. Wise JB, Witter SL: Argon laser therapy for open-angle glaucoma: a pilot study. *Arch Ophthalmol* 1979;97:319–322.
6. Thomas JV, Simmons RJ, Belcher CD III: Argon laser trabeculoplasty in the presurgical glaucoma patient. *Ophthalmology* 1982;89:187–197.
7. Wilensky JT, Jampol LM: Laser therapy for open-angle glaucoma. *Ophthalmology* 1981;88:213–217.
8. Robin AL, Pollack IP: Argon laser trabeculoplasty in secondary forms of open-angle glaucoma. *Arch Ophthalmol* 1983;101:382–384.
9. Schwartz AL, Perman KI, Whitten M: Argon laser trabeculoplasty in progressive low-tension glaucoma. *Ann Ophthalmol* 1984;16:560–566.
10. Krupin T, Patkin R, Kurata FK, Bishop KI, Keates EU, Kozart DM, Stone RA, Werner EB: Argon laser trabeculoplasty in black and white patients with primary open-angle glaucoma. *Ophthalmology* 1986;93:811–816.
11. Schwartz AL, Love DC, Schwartz MA: Long-term follow-up of argon laser trabeculoplasty for uncontrolled open-angle glaucoma. *Arch Ophthalmol* 1985;103:1482–1484.
12. Bishop KI, Krupin T, Feitl ME, Adelson A, Werner EB: Bilateral argon laser trabeculoplasty in primary open-angle glaucoma. *Am J Ophthalmol* 1989;107:591–595.
13. Melamed S, Pei J, Epstein DL: Delayed response to argon laser trabeculoplasty in monkeys: morphological and morphometric analysis. *Arch Ophthalmol* 1986;104:1078–1083.
14. Wise JB: Long-term control of adult open-angle glaucoma by argon laser treatment. *Ophthalmology* 1981;88:197–202.
15. Bylsma SS, Samples JR, Acott TS, Van Buskirk EM: Trabecular cell division after argon laser trabeculoplasty. *Arch Ophthalmol* 1988;106:544–547.
16. Melamed S, Pei J, Epstein DL: Short-term effect of argon laser trabeculoplasty in monkeys. *Arch Ophthalmol* 1985;103:1546–1552.
17. Van Buskirk EM, Pond V, Rosenquist RC, Acott TS: Argon laser trabeculoplasty: studies of mechanism of action. *Ophthalmology* 1984;91:1005–1010.
18. Rouhiainen HJ, Terasvirta ME, Tuovinen EJ: Peripheral anterior synechiae formation after trabeculoplasty. *Arch Ophthalmol* 1988;106:189–191.
19. Rodrigues MM, Spaeth GL, Donohoo P: Electron microscopy of argon therapy in phakic open-angle glaucoma. *Ophthalmology* 1982;89:198–210.
20. Weinreb RN, Ruderman J, Juster R, Zweig K: Immediate intraocular pressure response to argon laser trabeculoplasty. *Am J Ophthalmol* 1983;95:279–286.
21. Hoskins HD, Hetherington J, Minckler DS, Lieberman MF, Shaffer RN: Complications of laser trabeculoplasty. *Ophthalmology* 1983;90:796–799.
22. Greenidge KC, Rodrigues MM, Spaeth GL, Traverso CE, Weinreb S: Acute intraocular pressure elevation after argon laser trabeculoplasty and iridectomy: a clinicopathologic study. *Ophthalmic Surg* 1984;15:105–110.
23. Weinreb RN, Weaver D, Mitchell MD: Prostanoids in rabbit aqueous humor: effect

of laser photocoagulation of the iris. *Invest Ophthalmol Vis Sci* 1985;26:1087–1092.

24. Weinreb RN, Ruderman J, Juster R, Wilensky JT: Influence of the number of laser burns administered on the early results of argon laser trabeculoplasty. *Am J Ophthalmol* 1983;95:287–292.

25. Ofner S, Samples JR, Van Buskirk EM: Pilocarpine and the increase in intraocular pressure after trabeculoplasty. *Am J Ophthalmol* 1984;97:647–649.

26. Robin AL, Pollack IP, House B, Enger C: Effects of ALO 2145 on intraocular pressure following argon laser trabeculoplasty. *Arch Ophthalmol* 1987;105:646–650.

27. Thoming C, Van Buskirk EM, Samples JR: The corneal endothelium after laser therapy for glaucoma. *Am J Ophthalmol* 1987;103:518–522.

28. Moulin F, Haut J, Rached JA: Late failures of trabeculoplasty. *Int Ophthalmol* 1987; 10:61–66.

29. Shingleton BJ, Richter CU, Bellows AR, Hutchinson BT, Glynn RJ: Long-term efficacy of argon laser trabeculoplasty. *Ophthalmology* 1987;94:1513–1518.

30. Starita RJ, Fellman RL, Spaeth GL, Poryzees E: The effect of repeating full-circumference argon laser trabeculoplasty. *Ophthalmic Surg* 1984;15:41–43.

31. Brown SVL, Thomas JV, Simmons RJ: Laser trabeculoplasty re-treatment. *Am J Ophthalmol* 1985;99:8–10.

32. Messner D, Siegel LI, Kass MA, Kolker AE, Gordon M: Repeat argon laser trabeculoplasty. *Am J Ophthalmol* 1987;103:113–115.

33. Jorizzo PA, Samples JR, Van Buskirk EM: The effect of repeat argon laser trabeculoplasty. *Am J Ophthalmol* 1988;106:682–685.

CHAPTER 14

Laser Cyclophotocoagulation

Wallace L. M. Alward

- Introduction
- Transpupillary Cyclophotocoagulation
- Endophotocoagulation
- Transscleral Cyclophotocoagulation
  Noncontact Nd:YAG Cyclophotocoagulation
  Contact Nd:YAG Cyclophotocoagulation
  Other Lasers
- References

INTRODUCTION

Most surgical procedures for glaucoma are designed to increase aqueous outflow. Operations to decrease aqueous production destroy portions of the ciliary body and have many potential complications. These procedures generally are reserved for those situations in which techniques to enhance outflow are not possible or have not been successful. Cyclodestructive procedures frequently are used on eyes with neovascular, inflammatory, or aphakic glaucoma or on eyes with repeated failure of filtration surgery. These procedures also are useful to provide comfort for glaucomatous eyes with severe vision loss.

Cyclodiathermy was introduced by Weve in 1933[1] and popularized by Vogt in 1936.[2] This procedure had associated phthisis, uveitis, hemorrhage, and scleral necrosis.[3] Bietti described cyclocryotherapy using dry ice in 1950.[3] Bellows and Grant found cyclocryotherapy to be effective in 59 percent of patients with a variety of glaucomas after 6 months of follow-up.[4] Of their patients with open-angle glaucoma, 77 percent were controlled after 6 months. Complications were found in 15.8 percent, including hypotony in 2 of 61 eyes. Others reported less success and more frequent complications. Krupin and coinvestigators performed 360 degree cyclocryotherapy on 50 eyes with neovascular glaucoma.[5] After a mean of 24.9 months, only 34 percent had well-controlled intraocular pressure. Of their group, 34 percent developed phthisis, and 58.5 percent of eyes with vision preoperatively ultimately lost light perception.

Cyclocryotherapy with nitrous oxide gas cooling remains the predominant form of ciliary body destruction used today. Alternatives to cyclocryotherapy have been sought because of complications, which include pain,

159

postoperative pressure rise, inflammation, and hypotony. Other means of ciliary body destruction have included beta irradiation,[6] cycloelectrolysis,[7] xenon light coagulation,[8] therapeutic ultrasound,[9] and partial excision of the ciliary body.[10,11] More recently, laser energy has been used to cause ciliary body damage and decrease aqueous production.

Three principal routes of administering laser energy to the ciliary body have been employed: transpupillary cyclophotocoagulation, endophotocoagulation, and transscleral cyclophotocoagulation.

TRANSPUPILLARY CYCLOPHOTOCOAGULATION

The transpupillary delivery of argon green energy to the ciliary body was first described in rabbits by Lee in 1971.[12] Merritt, in 1976, reported on seven human eyes treated with transpupillary cyclophotocoagulation.[13] The laser energy was delivered through a Goldmann three-mirror lens using scleral depression to bring the ciliary processes into view. Although the majority of Merritt's eyes had a transient decrease in intraocular pressure, only one of seven had a long-lasting intraocular pressure reduction. In 1979, Lee described 14 aphakic patients who had a decrease in intraocular pressure directly related to the number of processes treated.[14] The patients' eyes were maximally dilated and anesthetized with topical agents. Through a goniolens, argon blue-green energy was administered in 50 to 100 μm spot sizes at 1 W of power for a duration of 0.1 to 0.2 sec. Eight to twenty-seven processes were treated in one to four treatments. In Lee's study, 71 percent of eyes showed a decrease in intraocular pressure.[14] Complications were uncommon and consisted of a mild punctate epitheliopathy and iridocyclitis. Mild bleeding from the ciliary processes was noted in one eye. Lee believed that at least one quarter of the ciliary body must be treated for an adequate reduction in intraocular pressure.

Transpupillary cyclophotocoagulation is a valuable treatment modality to consider in the few eyes in which an adequate transpupillary view of the ciliary body can be obtained (Table 14–1). The technique requires a large pupil

---

TABLE 14–1. Transpupillary Cyclophotocoagulation

Spot Size	50–200 μm
Duration	0.1—0.2 sec
Power	700–1000 mW
Wavelength	Argon blue-green
Contact Lens	Goldmann three-mirror
Anesthesia	Topical

Goal: To ablate 90–180 degrees of the ciliary body.

Note: The pupil is maximally dilated. Treatment is administered through a Goldmann three-mirror lens using scleral depression with a cotton-tipped applicator to bring the ciliary processes into view. The power is increased until the ciliary processes demonstrate whitening and shrinkage. All visible processes in one or two quadrants are treated. Postoperatively, the eye is treated with topical corticosteroids and cycloplegics. The corticosteroids and cycloplegics are tapered gradually as inflammation resolves.

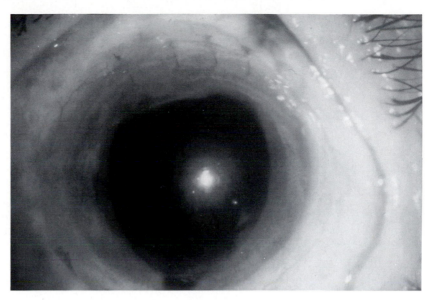

Figure 14–1. Gonioscopic view of transpupillary cyclophotocoagulation in a patient with traumatic aniridia. Note the whitening of the treated ciliary processes.

and a clear cornea. Even if the anterior ciliary body processes are visible, it can be difficult to adequately destroy the posterior portion of the ciliary body processes from this approach.[15] It is a technique worth considering in eyes with congenital or traumatic aniridia (Fig. 14–1) and in aphakic eyes with large sector iridectomies.

ENDOPHOTOCOAGULATION

Shields and co-workers, in 1985, described pressure lowering after endophotocoagulation of the ciliary body in monkeys.[15] In 1986, Patel and co-workers employed argon laser endophotocoagulation after vitrectomy in 18 human eyes.[16] The laser probe was introduced through the pars plana and was placed 2 to 4 mm from the ciliary body processes. A cotton-tipped applicator was used to indent the sclera to bring ciliary processes into view through the pupil. A power of 500 to 700 mW was applied for 0.5 to 1.0 sec. An area of 150 to 360 degrees was treated, usually 240 degrees. They found the intraocular pressure to be lowered in 14 of 18 eyes. Of the 18 patients treated in their study, only 1 developed postoperative hypotony. Inflammation and pain were thought to be less severe than with cyclocryotherapy. Shields reported using a shorter duration (0.2 sec) with more power (1000 mW).[17] He treated each process in two quadrants, with three to five applications of laser energy to each process.

Transvitreal endophotocoagulation is employed in aphakic eyes or in eyes that are undergoing lensectomy at the time of the operation (Table 14–2). Patel recommends vitrectomy to decrease the chance of complications caused by extensive intraocular manipulation of the anterior vitreous. It is a more involved and invasive procedure than the transpupillary or transscleral approaches. One should remember this procedure for those patients with uncontrolled glaucoma who are undergoing vitrectomy for other reasons, such as diabetics with neovascular glaucoma who are undergoing vitrectomy for hemorrhage.

TABLE 14–2. Endophotocoagulation

Spot Size	Fixed 20-gauge probe
Duration	0.2—1.0 sec
Power	500–1000 mW
Wavelength	Argon blue-green
Contact Lens	None
Anesthesia	Retrobulbar

Goal: To ablate 180–240 degrees of the ciliary body.

Note: The pupil is maximally dilated. Under retrobulbar anesthesia, a pars plana vitrectomy and, if needed, lensectomy are performed. Ciliary processes are brought into view by depressing the sclera with a cotton-tipped applicator. A 20-gauge fiberoptic probe is positioned 2–4 mm from the ciliary body. The laser power is adjusted until the ciliary processes whiten, shrink, and form a central pit. Postoperatively, subconjunctival antibiotics and corticosteroids are administered. Topical antibiotics, corticosteroids, and atropine are used and gradually tapered.[15,17]

TRANSSCLERAL CYCLOPHOTOCOAGULATION

Of the three approaches to laser destruction of the ciliary body, transscleral Nd:YAG cyclophotocoagulation has become the most widely adopted. Because the energy is delivered through the sclera, this approach is not limited to eyes with clear corneas and large pupils, as the transpupillary technique is. The transscleral technique is not as invasive as endophotocoagulation.

As in cyclocryotherapy, transscleral cyclophotocoagulation is performed through intact conjunctiva and sclera. Transscleral use of the polychromatic xenon light was first used by Weekers and co-workers, who suggested that the light would pass through the nonpigmented conjunctiva and sclera and be absorbed by pigmented ciliary body.[8] Weekers discovered that when enough energy was delivered to cause a decrease in intraocular pressure, there were marked side effects, such as iritis and hyphema.

Beckman and colleagues, in 1972, delivered pulsed ruby laser energy transsclerally.[18] Although effective, this technique never gained wide use, partly due to lack of availability of the laser.[19]

More recently, the continuous wave Nd:YAG energy has been employed. The Nd:YAG laser emits light in the infrared region of the spectrum (1064 nm). Light at this wavelength penetrates the sclera six times more readily than does argon blue-green light.[20] Beckman and Sugar first reported the use of the neodymium laser on humans in 1973.[21] They had successful lowering of intraocular pressure in 13 of 18 eyes treated (using intraocular pressure of ≤30 mm Hg as a definition of success). The commercial availability of continuous wave Nd:YAG lasers in the mid-1980s generated studies on this mode of ciliary body destruction. In 1985, Nd:YAG photocoagulation in rabbits was shown to create visible burns of the ciliary body and caused reduction of intraocular pressure.[19] Studies on human autopsy eyes grossly[22] and histopathologically[23] led to the development of current treatment parameters. Transscleral Nd:YAG cyclophotocoagulation seems to have less associated pain, inflammation, visual loss, and early intraocular pressure rise than has cyclocryotherapy.[24]

Continuous wave Nd:YAG laser can be delivered through either contact or noncontact systems. The only instrument available for noncontact Nd:YAG cyclophotocoagulation is the LASAG Microruptor. There are several contact continuous wave Nd:YAG lasers available. It is important to recognize that a standard Q-switched Nd:YAG laser generally is incapable of continuous wave output.

Noncontact Nd:YAG Cyclophotocoagulation

Noncontact Nd:YAG laser energy is administered via a slit-lamp delivery system, with or without a contact lens (Table 14–3) (Fig. 14–2). The contact lens described by Shields compresses the conjunctiva and blanches blood vessels.[25] It is believed that this lens standardizes the depth of conjunctiva through which the beam passes and provides smaller, more rapidly healing, conjunctival burns. It also holds the lids apart.

Hampton and coauthors reported a series of 100 patients treated with the LASAG Microruptor II.[24] They used a duration of 20 msec with an energy level of 7 to 8 J. The Nd:YAG beam was offset to be focused deeper than the helium-neon aiming beam (setting 9 on the LASAG Microruptor II). The treatment was delivered to the conjunctiva 1.0 to 1.5 mm from the limbus, being farther from the limbus in the superior and inferior quadrants and closer in the nasal and temporal quadrants. They applied laser energy to 28 to 32 spots over 360 degrees. Subconjunctival steroids and topical atropine were administered at the conclusion of the procedure, and the patient was maintained on topical atropine and corticosteroids or a corticosteroid–antibiotic combination.

A study comparing treatments performed 1.5 mm from the limbus with those performed 3.0 mm from the limbus found better intraocular pressure lowering in the eyes treated closer to the limbus.[26]

In a study of 106 eyes of 100 patients, Hampton and associates reported a success rate of 51 percent after the first treatment. They defined success as an intraocular pressure of 7 to 20 mm Hg with or without medication. A qualified success was defined as an intraocular pressure ≤ 7 mm Hg or ≥ 20 mm Hg but requiring no further surgery. Seventeen percent of patients were clas-

---

TABLE 14–3. Noncontact Nd:YAG Transscleral Cyclophotocoagulation

Spot Size	Fixed 70 μm
Duration	20 msec
Energy	4–8 J
Wavelength	Continuous wave Nd:YAG
Contact Lens	None or shields
Anesthesia	Retrobulbar

Goal: To treat the ciliary body over 360 degrees with 28–32 applications of Nd:YAG energy.

Note: After retrobulbar anesthesia, the patient is brought to the slit lamp at the laser. The Nd:YAG laser is used in a free-running thermal mode. The Nd:YAG laser energy is offset to be focused deeper than the helium-neon aiming beam. On the LASAG laser, the offset is set at 9 (3.6 mm in air).[24] The energy is focused 1 mm from the limbus nasally and temporally and 1.5 mm from the limbus superiorly and inferiorly.[24] After 28–32 applications, subconjunctival corticosteroids are administered, and the eye is patched. Postoperatively, the eye is treated with topical corticosteroids and a topical cycloplegic. These postoperative drops are tapered as inflammation subsides.

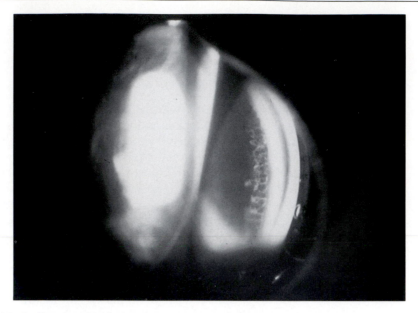

Figure 14–2. Transscleral Nd:YAG cyclophotocoagulation. Note that the laser applications are administered approximately 1.5 mm posterior to the limbus.

sified as qualified successes. Thirty-two percent were classified as failures. Of the 32 failures, 29 required more Nd:YAG cyclophotocoagulation, 1 had subsequent cyclocryotherapy, 1 had a retrobulbar alcohol injection, and 1 was enucleated. Success was more likely if the patient was older and if the patient had a lower preoperative intraocular pressure.[24]

In the study by Hampton and colleagues, a rise in intraocular pressure of 3 to 30 mm Hg was noted in 22 percent of patients at 1 to 2 hours (mean of 10.8 mm Hg). At 1 day, 9 percent of patients had an intraocular pressure that had elevated by 3 to 15 mm Hg (mean of 8.3 mm Hg). Visual acuity decreased in 27 of the 65 patients with intraocular pressure control after one or more treatments. Vision loss, the most common complication, was from a variety of causes. A recognized cause of vision loss, such as corneal edema or cataract, could be found in 51 percent of those losing vision. Other complications included severe inflammation in 29 percent, severe pain in 12 percent, and hyphema in 8 percent. Five pseudophakic patients developed posterior capsule opacification, three patients developed graft rejection, two patients developed cataract, and one had a vitreous hemorrhage.[24]

Contact Nd:YAG Cyclophotocoagulation:

Contact transscleral continuous wave Nd:YAG laser cyclophotocoagulation is more readily available than noncontact. The equipment is less expensive than that used for noncontact Nd:YAG laser. Additionally, the contact Nd:YAG laser has applications in fields other than ophthalmology and is available in many hospitals. Whereas noncontact Nd:YAG laser cyclophotocoagulation is delivered through a slit lamp to a seated patient, the contact Nd:YAG laser is delivered through a fiberoptic cable to a supine patient. This enables the surgeon to treat children and others under general anesthesia. Contact Nd:YAG laser cyclophotocoagulation uses lower energy levels and longer exposures than the noncontact technique (Table 14–4). This produces a coagulative necrosis of the ciliary body rather than the blistering seen with noncontact Nd:YAG laser cyclophotocoagulation. This may be the reason that this procedure seems to have less associated pain, inflammation, and vision loss.[27]

TABLE 14–4. Contact Nd:YAG Transscleral Cyclophotocoagulation

Spot Size	Fixed tip diameter
Duration	0.5–0.7 sec
Power	4–9 W
Wavelength	Continuous wave Nd:YAG
Contact Lens	None
Anesthesia	Retrobulbar

Goal: To damage the ciliary body and decrease aqueous production.

Note: Retrobulbar anesthesia is administered. The laser is set at about 7 W with a duration of 0.7 sec. The sapphire tip is placed with the anterior portion 0.5–1.5 mm from the limbus. Thirty to forty applications are delivered around the circumference, sparing 3 and 9 o'clock. Subconjunctival corticosteroids are administered, and the eye is patched for several hours. A tapering schedule of topical corticosteroids and cycloplegics is instituted.

The Nd:YAG energy is delivered through a quartz fiber to a synthetic sapphire tip. The tip is placed on the conjunctiva over the ciliary body with the anterior edge 0.5 to 1.5 mm from the limbus. Four to nine watts of energy are used for a duration of 0.5 to 0.7 sec. The entire circumference of the ciliary body is treated with 30 to 40 spots. Some authors recommend leaving the 3 o'clock and the 9 o'clock areas untreated to avoid damage to the long posterior ciliary arteries.[27] When 7 W and 9 W of power were compared, they were found to cause similar amounts of lowering of intraocular pressure. The higher power was associated with more frequent inflammation and complications.[27]

In a study of 140 eyes treated with contact Nd:YAG cyclophotocoagulation, the mean drop in intraocular pressure was 16.8 mm Hg (44 percent).[27] Eyes with higher preoperative intraocular pressures tended to have higher postoperative intraocular pressures. The onset of maximum intraocular pressure reduction was 1 week to 1 month. Early postoperative intraocular pressure spikes were not common. An increase in intraocular pressure of more than 8 mm Hg was seen in 9 percent of eyes at 1 hour and 6 percent of eyes at 1 day. Patients did not often have substantial pain after this procedure. Postoperative inflammation was seen but is less than with cyclocryotherapy. Vision loss occurred in 7 percent, and 2 eyes were enucleated for persistent pain.

Other Lasers

Other lasers have been tried transsclerally. Argon and krypton lasers caused minimal and transient intraocular pressure lowering in rabbits and monkeys. These wavelengths also caused thermal damage to the sclera.[28] Contact transscleral cyclophotocoagulation with a semiconductor diode laser has been described in rabbits.[29]

REFERENCES

1. Weve H: Die Zyklodiatermie das corpus ciliare bei Glaukom. *Zentralbl Ophthalmol* 1933;29:562–569.
2. Vogt A: Versuche zue intraokularen Druckherabsetzung mittelst Diathermieschädigung des Corpus ciliare. *Klin Monatstbl Aufenjeilkd* 1936;97:672–677.

3. Bietti G: Surgical intervention of the ciliary body. *JAMA* 1950;142:889–897.
4. Bellows AR, Grant WM: Cyclocryotherapy in advanced inadequately controlled glaucoma. *Am J Ophthalmol* 1973;75:679–684.
5. Krupin T, Mitchell KB, Becker B: Cyclocryotherapy in neovascular glaucoma. *Am J Ophthalmol* 1978;86:24–26.
6. Haik GM, Breffeilh LA, Barbar A: Beta irradiation as a possible therapeutic agent in glaucoma. *Am J Ophthalmol* 1948;31:945–952.
7. Berens C, Sheppard LB, Duel AB: Cycloelectrolysis for glaucoma. *Trans Am Ophthalmol Soc* 1949;47:364–380.
8. Weekers R, Lavergne G, Watillon M, Gilson M, Legros AM: Effects of photocoagulation of ciliary body upon ocular tension. *Am J Ophthalmol* 1961;52:156–163.
9. Burgess SEP, Silverman RH, Coleman DJ, Yablonski ME, Lizzi FL, Driller J, Rosado A, Dennis PH: Treatment of glaucoma with high-intensity focused ultrasound. *Ophthalmology* 1986;93:831–838.
10. Freyler H, Scheimbauer I: Excision of the ciliary body (Sautter procedure) as a last resort in secondary glaucoma. *Klin Monatsbl Augenheikld* 1981;179:473–477.
11. Demeler U: Ciliary surgery for glaucoma. *Trans Ophthalmol Soc UK* 1986;105:242–245.
12. Lee P-F, Pomerantzeff O: Transpupillary cyclophotocoagulation of rabbit eyes. *Am J Ophthalmol* 1971;71:911–920.
13. Merritt JC: Transpupillary photocoagulation of the ciliary processes. *Ann Ophthalmol* 1976;8:325–328.
14. Lee P-F: Argon laser photocoagulation of the ciliary processes in cases of aphakic glaucoma. *Arch Ophthalmol* 1979;97:2135–2138.
15. Shields B, Chandler DB, Hickingbotham D, Klintworth GK: Intraocular cyclophotocoagulation. *Arch Ophthalmol* 1985;103:1731–1735.
16. Patel A, Thompson JT, Michels RG, Quigley HA: Endolaser treatment of the ciliary body for uncontrolled glaucoma. *Ophthalmology* 1986;93:825–830.
17. Shields MB: Cyclodestructive surgery for glaucoma: past, present, and future. *Trans Am Acad Ophthalmol Otolaryngol* 1985;83:285–303.
18. Beckman H, Kinoshita A, Rota AN, Sugar HS: Transscleral ruby laser irradiation of the ciliary body in the treatment of intractable glaucoma. *Trans Am Acad Ophthalmol Otolaryngol* 1972;76:423–436.
19. Wilensky JT, Welch D, Mirolovich M: Transscleral cyclophotocoagulation using a neodymium: YAG laser. *Ophthalmic Surg* 1985;16:95–98.
20. Van Der Zypen E, Fankhauser F: Lasers in the treatment of chronic simple glaucoma. *Trans Ophthal Soc UK* 1982;102:147–153.
21. Beckman H, Sugar HS: Neodymium laser cyclophotocoagulation. *Arch Ophthalmol* 1973;90:27–28.
22. Fankhauser F, van der Zypen E, Kwasniewska S, Rol P, England C: Transscleral cyclophotocoagulation using a neodymium YAG laser. *Ophthalmic Surg* 1986;17:94–100.
23. Hampton C, Shields MB: Transscleral neodymium-YAG cyclophotocoagulation—a histologic study of human autopsy eyes. *Arch Ophthalmol* 1988;106:1121–1123.
24. Hampton C, Shields MB, Miller KN, Blasini M: Evaluation of a protocol for transscleral neodymium: YAG cyclophotocoagulation in one hundred patients. *Ophthalmology* 1990;97:910–917.
25. Shields MB, Blasini M, Simmons R, Erickson PJ: A contact lens for transscleral Nd:YAG cyclophotocoagulation. *Am J Ophthalmol* 1989;108:457–458.
26. Crymes BM, Gross RL: Laser placement in noncontact Nd:YAG cyclophotocoagulation. *Am J Ophthalmol* 1990;110:670–673.
27. Schuman JS, Puliafito CA, Allingham RR, Belcher CD, Bellows AR, Latina MA, Shingleton BJ: Contact transscleral continuous wave neodymium: YAG laser cyclophotocoagulation. *Ophthalmology* 1990;97:571–580.
28. Peyman GA, Conway MD, Raichand M, Lin J: Histopathologic studies on transscleral argon-krypton photocoagulation with an exolaser probe. *Ophthalmic Surg* 1984;15:496–501.
29. Schuman JS, Jacobson JJ, Puliafito C, Noecker RJ, Reidy WT: Experimental use of semiconductor diode laser in contact transscleral cyclophotocoagulation in rabbits. *Arch Ophthalmol* 1990;108:1152–1157.

CHAPTER 15

YAG Laser Capsulotomy

Hansjoerg E. Kolder

- **Introduction**
- **Indications**
- **Laser Treatment**
  YAG Laser Setup
  Power Setting
  Complications During Procedure
  Follow-up
  Postoperative Complications
- **References**

INTRODUCTION

This chapter deals with the use of the yttrium-aluminum-garnet (YAG) laser to perform a capsulotomy.[1–8] Other applications are possible, for example, iridotomy, membranotomy, and cyclophotocoagulation, but are not dealt with specifically.[9–17] Recent developments, such as an erbium: YAG laser or compact diode lasers, have to await proof of their usefulness for capsulotomies. Several publications contain practical suggestions for the use of YAG lasers.[18–21]

The neodymium: YAG (Nd:YAG) solid state laser uses a synthetic crystal in which some yttrium ions are replaced by the element neodymium.[22,23] The wavelength of the YAG laser is 1064 nm, corresponding to invisible, near infrared radiation. The laser is pumped by a flash bulb, and the heat is removed by air or water cooling. An electrooptical crystal of high quality switches the YAG laser to produce pulses. Therefore, the laser is referred to as Q-switched. Such a laser pulse lasts nanoseconds (10^{-9} sec). Shorter pulses in picoseconds (10^{-12} sec) are obtained by a mode-locking device that selects frequencies.

The energy (in millijoule) delivered by currently available ophthalmic YAG lasers can be varied up to 10 mJ or more. The density of a laser beam is given as energy per area, but the spot size of an ophthalmic YAG laser usually is fixed and measures about 25 μm (10^{-6}m) in diameter.

Q-switched and mode-locked lasers produce an optical breakdown when focused within a transparent medium.[24,25] Low-energy pulses are transmitted through such media, and high-energy density opacifies transparent tissue, accompanied by a spark and sound. At this moment a physical plasma is formed consisting of electrons and ions. The plasma heats up and expands rapidly, which in turn creates a shockwave, initially at supersonic speed. The expanding plasma leaves a gas bubble behind.

The tissue disruption is dependent on the angle of convergence, usually 16 degrees, and the homogeneity of the laser mode (minimizing optical aberrations). The size of the tissue disruption can be increased by raising the energy of each pulse or by delivering several pulses in bursts.

The YAG laser requires a slit lamp and an aiming system consisting of an independent helium-neon (He-Ne) red laser. The patient should be seated comfortably and avoid movements. Neither topical anesthesia nor retrobulbar akinesia are routinely required. A contact lens sometimes is necessary to stabilize the patient's eye, increase the angle of incidence, and magnify the target.

INDICATIONS

An anterior capsulotomy before a planned extracapsular cataract extraction may facilitate the subsequent extracapsular cataract extraction by hydration of the cortex. A time interval of several hours has been reported between anterior capsulotomy and lens extraction. The uncertainty of the degree of cortical hydration, an inflammatory response, and improved techniques for anterior capsulotomy, like the can-opener maneuver, capsulorhexis, and ultrasonic-assisted capsulotomy, have reduced or eliminated the need for staged YAG laser anterior capsulotomies.

The YAG laser posterior capsulotomy has become the accepted and widely available technique for opening an opacified posterior capsule in aphakic or pseudophakic eyes.[26] Argon laser energy is not well absorbed by the posterior capsule. The alternative, a discission by needle or needle knife, sometimes is necessary for especially thick posterior capsules or when a primary posterior capsulotomy is indicated intraoperatively. Posterior capsules also can be removed incidental to a vitrectomy.

Vitreous strands, anterior capsular shreds distorting the pupil, and zonular fibers attached to the incision represent other indications for the use of a YAG laser, as does an opacified anterior lens capsule either inadvertently adherent to an intraocular lens in the pupil or an intentionally created small anterior capsulotomy that impedes subsequently the visualization for treatment of retinal disorders.

When a posterior capsule opacification develops, the patient complains about decreased visual acuity, glare, loss of contrast sensitivity, or photophobia. Retinoscopy is possible, but neither pinhole nor a new manifest refraction improves the visual acuity. Slit-lamp examination with side illumination may show folds in the posterior capsule or a fibrillar structure. This view also permits identification of an empty space behind the posterior capsule and in front of the vitreous face, if these structures have separated. The most important diagnostic aid for identification of an opacified posterior capsule is retroillumination through the slit lamp. Viewing the capsule binocularly in retroillumination permits an estimate of its thickness. Sometimes the posterior capsule appears uniform in retroillumination but has a quality of irregularity and thickness that can be confirmed with side illumination. Frequently, though, the opacified posterior capsule manifests itself by a vesicular pattern, suggestive of the formation of flattened Elschnig pearls. Significant condensation of vitreous may be observed behind the posterior capsule but is difficult to remove with the YAG laser.

The incidence of posterior capsule opacification varies with the time since cataract extraction and possibly with the configuration of the posterior surface of the implant lens and the vigor with which the posterior capsule has been polished. Phacoemulsification or planned extracapsular nuclear expression are followed by the same incidence of opacified posterior capsules. About 40 percent of posterior capsules develop visually significant opacifications within 5 years postoperatively. The incidence of an opacified posterior capsule seems unrelated to the age of the patient if one disregards the almost universal postoperative capsular opacification in children.

The indications for a YAG laser capsulotomy follow those for a cataract extraction: impairment of visual function interfering with the patient's visual needs. Since a YAG laser capsulotomy carries no risk of infection or expulsive hemorrhage and only a small risk for blindness[27] and for corneal decompensation, the major concerns in considering risk vs benefit are the transient intraocular pressure increase[28-31] and the development of a retinal tear caused by the contraction of vitreous strands.[32,33] A phototoxic effect on the retina is unlikely.[34,35] About one third of patients who undergo a posterior capsulotomy will experience a pressure increase of 8 mm Hg or more during the first 24 hours after laser treatment. Untreated, the pressure may rise to 40 mm Hg or higher and cause considerable discomfort. The pressure usually can be controlled by topical beta-blocking medication. The incidence of a retinal tear with retinal detachment is less than 1 percent after YAG capsulotomy. No preventive measure has been devised to decrease the incidence of retinal detachments. Low power of the YAG laser, waiting for the separation of the vitreous face from the posterior capsule, and some designs of the posterior surface of the implant lens may be beneficial. With the reintroduction of extracapsular cataract extraction in the early 1970s, some surgeons advocated a "preventive posterior capsulotomy" at the time of cataract extraction or soon afterward. However, the incidence of retinal detachments proved to be unacceptably high. The preferred time interval between cataract extraction and posterior capsulotomy is now 3 months or longer.

LASER TREATMENT

YAG Laser Setup

The YAG laser delivery system consists of a cooled laser module and a slit lamp (Table 15–1). Warmup time for the equipment is minimal. The optical delivery system has safeguards to prevent the reflected laser beam from reaching the operator's eye. The laser delivery system includes a standby mode in which the equipment should remain unless actually in use.

The preparation of the patient should include an explanation of the procedure, a short description of the focusing mechanism, how the laser removes the opacified posterior capsule, and a statement that the YAG laser capsulotomy is a definitive procedure preventing another cataract. Informed consent is required explaining the risks. A brief review of the patient's medical history should be documented, and comorbid conditions should be addressed. The patient should be informed that the laser beam is invisible, but the aiming light is red and that an afterimage may persist for a few seconds after the treatment. The patient should be seated comfortably in front of the slit lamp. Adjustments are important for the height of the chair, the chin rest, and support for the arms. No anesthesia is required. For some patients who find it difficult to fixate, a contact lens is necessary and is inserted after topical anesthesia. Some slit lamps provide a band to fasten around the patient's head. If used, its purpose should be explained carefully to the patient to avoid anxiety from the restraint. Patients with breathing difficulties should be encouraged to interrupt breathing briefly before laser energy is delivered. Mydriasis is necessary to establish the extent of the capsule opacification, but laser energy can be delivered through an undilated pupil.

The midpupillary area is the best starting point for the capsulotomy. The posterior capsule should be visible in side illumination or retroillumination.

TABLE 15–1. YAG Posterior Capsulotomy

Initial Power Setting	0.8 mJ
Initial Pulse Setting	Single
Contact Lens	Usually not needed
Anesthesia	Usually not needed

Goal: To create a central opening in the opacified posterior capsule to improve the patient's vision and to facilitate subsequent fundus examinations.

Note: Use broad, dim, side illumination or retroillumination with 25× magnification. Laser treatment can be performed with or without mydriasis. The patient should be instructed as to the color and sound of the laser treatment. Adequate tear maintenance is important. It is important to minimize reflection and adjust the intensity of the aiming beam. Synchronizing triggering of the YAG laser with respiratory and circulatory movement of the patient may be helpful. The two aiming beams are adjusted posterior to the lens capsule, and the slit lamp is then moved toward the capsule until the two aiming beams overlap. Single shots varying in intensity between 0.8 and 2.5 mJ are administered, and bursts of pulses are used if necessary. The effect of each application is assessed. Once the posterior capsule is penetrated, observe the direction of the split and follow the split with shots until the opening is central and about 4 mm in diameter. The total number of applications should be limited to 30 or less per treatment session. Visual acuity and intraocular pressure are measured 1 hour posttreatment.

Some instruments provide a separate joystick for manipulation of the aiming beam. Focusing is crucial for laser treatment. The double aiming beam (He-Ne) should be focused initially posterior to the capsule so that two spots are visible on the capsule. The slit lamp is then slowly moved toward the opacified capsule until the two aiming beams fuse. At that moment, the laser energy will be concentrated on the posterior capsule. Optical corrections are built into the instrument such that the invisible, infrared laser beam is focused on the same spot as the visible, red He-Ne aiming beams. A compromise has to be found between the patient's being advised not to blink and the deterioration of imagery caused by drying of the cornea. It is advisable to give the patient a rest period with eyelid closure every 10 to 15 sec to prevent image deterioration. These precautions are not necessary if a contact lens is used, but the contact lens per se may induce corneal edema.

Power Setting

After setting up the equipment, a dry run should be performed by taping a piece of paper in the place where the patient's eye will be. The low laser energy (1 mJ) required to produce a capsular opening will not mark the paper, but a setting of 10 mJ or a burst of 10 pulses delivering 1 mJ each will mark the paper and give evidence of the effectiveness of the instrument. The energy is measured internally, and the calibration is factory set. The initial setting for a posterior YAG laser capsulotomy should be 1 mJ or less. The spot size is invariant. Frequently, it is not necessary to deliver bursts of pulses. When YAG lasers first came into use, the goal was to produce a large capsulotomy opening. Different shapes were recommended, such as a D on its side. It was later realized that more energy favors the contraction of vitreous strands. At present, the least amount of laser energy is delivered that creates an adequate opening of 3 to 4 mm in diameter. A cross-pattern is useful. Depending on the tension within the posterior capsule, it is possible to effectuate a capsulotomy by using a single pulse in the pupillary center, to observe the formation of rents, and to enlarge the capsulotomy with a few more single pulses. While the capsulotomy appears initially irregular, it often rounds out and increases in size over time.[36] The energy required depends on the thickness of the posterior capsule. Rarely is it necessary to increase the energy per pulse to more than 2.5 mJ. Occasionally, bursts are more efficacious to create a hole. Some posterior capsules do not split and require repeated applications of YAG punctures to gradually enlarge the opening. The treatment should be interrupted after 30 to 50 applications of between 1 and 2.5 mJ. The intraocular pressure should be measured then, and the anterior chamber reaction should be observed. Subsequent enlargement of the capsulotomy should be planned accordingly.

Complications During Procedure

Positioning the patient comfortably is as important as adjustment of the oculars for the ophthalmologist and the proper combination of side and retroillumination to visualize the structure to be lasered. It has to be ascertained that the implant lens is not made of glass or, if so, that proper precautions are taken not to hit the implant lens because of the risk of shattering. Implant lenses that are hydrophobic, for example, silicone, may not develop adhesions in the capsular bag.[37] A capsulotomy may then cause the implant lens to dislocate posteriorly. At optical interfaces, such as the cornea or the anterior implant lens surface, reflections (Purkinje images) occur, impairing the visualization of the structure to be treated. Directing the patient's gaze slightly laterally reflects these Purkinje images off center. This can be accomplished by means of a fixation device incorporated into the slit lamp. No acoustic report is heard if therapeutic laser energy is delivered into an optically empty structure.

Laser energy imparted on the cornea causes a mark. No through and through track is produced because the large angle of incidence limits the depth of the laser lesion. Miss-aim on the iris is more likely if Purkinje images interfere with visualization. The patient may report pain, an iris puncture may be visible, or a hemorrhage may ensue. Such hemorrhage usually is confined to a trickle of erythrocytes floating down from the laser lesion. The hemorrhage rarely produces a layered hyphema, and frequently, laser treatment can be continued. The laser energy may unintentionally be delivered to the anterior or posterior surface of the implant lens. Polymethyl methacrylate (PMMA) lenses respond to laser energy with the formation of a small pit or fracture line. The former may not be easily visible. A crack is seen readily and may subtend a millimeter in length. It tends to remain localized. A laser mark in a silicone lens has the quality of a melted spot. It is imperative at such an occurrence to refocus the aiming beam and to be certain that two aiming spots are seen on the posterior capsule when the focus is in the vitreous and that one spot forms when the focus is moved toward the capsule. If YAG energy is delivered successfully to the posterior capsule, a break appears, which may run along a tension line. At this stage, the posterior capsule may separate from the posterior surface of the implant lens. If this happens, waiting a few seconds allows the surgeon to deliver laser energy farther away from the posterior surface of the implant lens, thereby reducing the risk of pitting. A fibrotic posterior capsule, such as a Soemmering's ring, will rarely split, and such a membrane has to be punctured with higher energy or bursts. Vitreous condensations do not split but can be punctured. They require considerably more energy to slowly burn the membrane away. The strategy for opening a membranous opacification consists of increasing the energy per pulse, up to about 2.5 mJ, and, if that does not suffice, to use bursts of pulses. When applying multiple pulses, the energy per pulse should be reduced. Careful observation of the treatment effect will guide the ophthalmologist to select the optimal combination of energy and number of pulses in a burst. Usually, increasing energy is more effective than doubling or tripling the pulses.

A laser beam aimed at the posterior surface of the implant lens may cause bubbles that may impede visualization of the posterior capsule. Waiting a few minutes allows the bubbles to rise. Bubbles are not indicative of a fracture line in the implant lens. The opacified posterior capsule should split with about 1 mJ of laser energy. If 2.5 mJ have no effect, a reassessment should be made about the appropriate aim and the thickness of the structure to be lasered. Occasionally, a needle knife discission has to supplant the YAG laser. A laser ridge or biconvex implant lens may slow the development of an opacification and alter the effect of a capsulotomy.[38]

Follow-up

The visual acuity should improve immediately after a YAG laser posterior capsulotomy, provided that an ametropia is corrected adequately. The intraocular pressure should be remeasured the following day if it needed treatment. Flare and an occasional cell rarely necessitate corticosteroid medication. A follow-up visit in 3 months is adequate, and the patient should be reassured that the YAG laser capsulotomy is a definitive procedure. If a patient experiences changes in vision, it is unlikely to be secondary to a reopacification of the posterior capsule. Other causes have to be explored, for example, cystoid macular edema, increased intraocular pressure, vitreous hemorrhage, or retinal detachment. Very rarely a patient can not tolerate a YAG laser procedure either because of infirmity, lack of cooperation at the slit lamp, or unavailability of a laser delivery system for treatment in the supine position. A needle knife capsulotomy is appropriate and effective in these cases.

Postoperative Complications

Iritis after a YAG laser capsulotomy manifests as flare or cellular reaction.[39] With fewer than 30 laser applications of 1 mJ, treatment of the iritis with topical steroids rarely is required. Occasionally, the eye of a diabetic patient will react with a massive outpouring of plasmoid aqueous that is, on first sight, indistinguishable from vitreous. Under such circumstances, frequent topical steroid medication and mydriasis are indicated.

The intraocular pressure may increase and should be measured approximately 1 hour after the procedure. An increase of 8 mm Hg above the preprocedure intraocular pressure should alert the ophthalmologist either to treat the patient with a beta-blocking agent, if not contraindicated, or to recheck the pressure an hour later. If headache or eye pain develops during the first 24 hours after the laser treatment, the patient should use an analgesic, such as acetaminophen 500 mg. If the pain is not relieved within 2 hours, the intraocular pressure has to be measured. Usually 1 drop of 0.5 percent timolol controls the pressure. Patients who have a pressure increase of more than 8 mm Hg and have received timolol are remeasured 1 hour later. If the pressure decreased during that hour, follow-up is arranged for the next day. In the future, apraclonidine may be approved as preprocedure medication.[40,41]

Implant lens pits may be recognized only during a postoperative visit. Glare or optical distortions from pits or fracture lines rarely are perceived by the patient. The capsulotomy opening may extend beyond the optics of the implant lens. Vitreous may then herniate immediately or with delay. A knuckle of vitreous in the anterior chamber rarely distorts the pupil. Vitreous face dehiscences occur frequently. A retinal detachment may develop after a

YAG laser capsulotomy in aphakic or pseudophakic eyes within a few days or after a delay of weeks or months. The patient should be instructed carefully about the symptoms of a retinal detachment and encouraged to seek attention should a flash of light occur, showers or floaters be observed, or a curtain obscure the vision.

Elschnig pearls behind an implant lens can best be seen in retroillumination. They can be penetrated adequately with YAG laser energy. Elschnig pearls outside the optical part of an implant lens cannot be treated successfully using the laser. They can be washed out but tend to reform. In an aphakic eye with exuberant Elschnig pearl formation, a surgical posterior capsulotomy is the definitive treatment.

For a fibrotic posterior capsule or vitreous condensation, a staggered YAG laser capsulotomy may be advisable. Thirty laser shots usually are well tolerated. Follow-up treatment can be applied as soon as it has been ascertained that the intraocular pressure did not rise significantly and that no plastic iritis has occurred. The edges of the capsulotomy opening may retract some over a period of a few days or weeks and make a secondary treatment unnecessary.

REFERENCES

1. Alpar JJ: Posterior capsulotomy in sulcus-fixated versus bag-fixated intraocular lenses in diabetic patients. *J Am Intraocul Implant Soc* 1985;11:577–580.
2. Axt JC: Nd:YAG laser posterior capsulotomy: a clinical study. *Am J Optom Physiol Opt* 1985;62:173–187.
3. Gimbel HV, Van Westenbrugge JA, Sanders DR, Raanan MG: Effect of sulcus vs capsular fixation of YAG-induced pressure rises following posterior capsulotomy. *Arch Ophthalmol* 1990;108:1126–1129.
4. McDonnell PJ, Zarbin MA, Green WR: Posterior capsule opacification in pseudophakic eyes. *Ophthalmology* 1983;90:1548–1553.
5. Sawusch MR, McDonnell PJ: Posterior capsule opacification. *Curr Opin Ophthalmol* 1990;1:2–7.
6. Steinert RF, Puliafito CA: YAG lasers in cataract surgery. *Int Ophthalmol Clin* 1987;27(3):181–194.
7. Terry AC, Stark WJ, Maumenee AE, Fagadau W: Neodymium-YAG laser for posterior capsulotomy. *Am J Ophthalmol* 1983;96:716–720.
8. Weiblinger RP: Review of the clinical literature on the use of the Nd:YAG laser for posterior capsulotomy. *J Cataract Refract Surg* 1986;12:162–170.
9. Alpar JJ: The role of 1% sodium hyaluronate in anterior capsulotomy with the neodymium:YAG laser in patients with diseased cornea. *J Cataract Refract Surg* 1986;12:658–661.
10. Bazard MC, Guldenfels Y, Raspiller A: Complications endothéliales précoces après traitement par laser néodymium-YAG. *J Fr Ophtalmol* 1989;12:17–23.
11. Crymes BM, Gross RL: Laser placement in noncontact Nd:YAG cyclophotocoagulation. *Am J Ophthalmol* 1990;110:670–673.
12. Geggel HS: Successful treatment of recurrent corneal erosion with Nd:YAG anterior stromal puncture. *Am J Ophthalmol* 1990;110:404–407.
13. Geyer O, Rothkoff L, Lazar M: Clearing of corneal argyrosis by YAG laser. *Br J Ophthalmol* 1989;73:1009–1010.
14. Krauss JM, Puliafito CA, Steinert RF: Laser interactions with the cornea. *Surv Ophthalmol* 1986;31:37–53.
15. Putterman AM: Scalpel neodymium:YAG laser in oculoplastic surgery. *Am J Ophthalmol* 1990;109:581–584.
16. Schubert HD, Agarwala A, Arbizo V: Changes in aqueous outflow after in vitro neodymium:yttrium aluminum garnet laser cyclophotocoagulation. *Invest Ophthalmol Vis Sci* 1990;31:1834–1838.
17. Trope GE, Ma S: Mid-term effects of neodymium:YAG transscleral cyclocoagulation in glaucoma. *Ophthalmology* 1990;97:73–75.
18. Deutsch TA, Goldberg MF: Neodymium:YAG laser capsulotomy. *Int Ophthalmol Clin* 1985;25(3):87–100.

19. Fankhauser F, Kwasniewska S, van der Zypen E: Die experimentelle und klinische Anwendung des im thermischen Betrieb arbeitenden Neodym:YAG Lasers. *Klin Mbl Augenheilk* 1987;191:169–173.
20. Fankhauser F, Rol P: Microsurgery with the neodymium:YAG laser: an overview. *Int Ophthalmol Clin* 1985;25(3):55–84.
21. March WF, ed. *Ophthalmology Clinics of North America, 2, Practical Laser Surgery*. Philadelphia: Saunders; 1989.
22. Loertscher H, Rol P: Basic physics of neodymium:YAG laser. *Int Ophthalmol Clin* 1985;25(3):1–14.
23. McCord RC: Neodymium:YAG laser: Theoretical and practical considerations. *Int Ophthalmol Clin* 1985;25(3):15–19.
24. Frankhauser F, Loertscher H, van der Zypen E: Clinical studies on high and low power laser radiation upon some structures of the anterior and posterior segments of the eye. Experiences in the treatment of some pathological conditions of the anterior and posterior segments of the human eye by means of a Nd:YAG laser, driven at various power levels. *Int Ophthalmol* 1982;5:15–32.
25. Zysset B, Fujimoto JG, Puliafito CA, Birngruber R, Deutsch TF: Picosecond optical breakdown: tissue effects and reduction of collateral damage. *Lasers Surg Med* 1989;9:193–204.
26. Liesegang TJ, Bourne WM, Ilstrup DM: Secondary surgical and neodymium-YAG laser discissions. *Am J Ophthalmol* 1985;100:510–519.
27. Blackwell C, Hirst LW, Kinnas SJ: Neodymium-YAG capsulotomy and potential blindness. *Am J Ophthalmol* 1984;98:521–522.
28. Ruderman JM, Mitchell PG, Kraff M: Pupillary block following Nd:YAG laser capsulotomy. *Ophthalmic Surg* 1983;14:418–419.
29. Schubert HD: A history of intraocular pressure rise with reference to the Nd:YAG laser. *Surv Ophthalmol* 1985;30:168–172.
30. Schubert HD: Vitreoretinal changes associated with rise in intraocular pressure after Nd:YAG capsulotomy. *Ophthalmic Surg* 1987;18:19–22.
31. Weinreb RN, Wasserstrom JP, Parker W: Neovascular glaucoma following neodymium-YAG laser posterior capsulotomy. *Arch Ophthalmol* 1986;104:730–731.
32. Koch DD, Liu JF, Gill EP, Parke DW II: Axial myopia increases the risk of retinal complications after neodymium-YAG laser posterior capsulotomy. *Arch Ophthalmol* 1989;107:986–990.
33. Ober RR, Wilkinson CP, Fiore JV Jr, Maggiano JM: Rhegmatogenous retinal detachment after neodymium-YAG laser capsulotomy in phakic and pseudophakic eyes. *Am J Ophthalmol* 1986;101:81–89.
34. Arneodo J, Azema A, Botineau J, Crozafon P: Illumination retinienne lors d'interventions au laser YAG picoseconde. *J Fr Ophthalmol* 1985;8:213–218.
35. Docchio F, Sacchi CA: Nd:YAG laser irradiation of an eye model: experimental analysis. *Lasers Surg Med* 1987;6:520–529.
36. Clayman HM, Jaffe NS: Spontaneous enlargement of neodymium:YAG posterior capsulotomy in aphakic and pseudophakic patients. *J Cataract Refract Surg* 1988;14:667–669.
37. Keates RH, Sall KN, Kreter JK: Effect of the Nd:YAG laser on polymethylmethacrylate, HEMA copolymer, and silicone intraocular materials. *J Cataract Refract Surg* 1987;13:401–409.
38. Story PG: Intraocular lenses with posterior convex optics: a clinical review. *Ophthalmic Surg* 1988;19:658–661.
39. Naveh N, Rosner M, Zborowsky-Gutman L, Rosen N, Weissman C: Comparison of the effects of argon and neodymium:YAG laser iridotomy on prostaglandin E_2 and blood–aqueous barrier disruption. *Ophthalmic Res* 1990;22:253–258.
40. Nesher R, Kolker AE: Delayed increased intraocular pressure after Nd:YAG laser posterior capsulotomy in a patient treated with apraclonidine. *Am J Ophthalmol* 1990;110:94–95.
41. Robin AL: Apraclonidine uses. *Arch Ophthalmol* 1990;108:337.

CHAPTER 16

Endophotocoagulation

Jose S. Pulido and Karen M. Joos

- ■ Introduction
- ■ Indications
- ■ Laser Treatment
  Optics
  Endolaser Operation
  Troubleshooting
- ■ References

Although the slit-lamp biomicroscope has become the most common laser delivery system in ophthalmology, two other methods are also widely used: (1) endolaser photocoagulation, which uses an intraocular fiberoptic probe, and (2) binocular indirect ophthalmoscopic systems. Many of the newer argon and krypton lasers can be adapted to allow these alternative modes of delivery.

INTRODUCTION

In 1979, Charles first described photocoagulation with an intraocular instrument powered by a portable xenon arc light.[1] The technique proved to be an extremely useful intraoperative alternative to diathermy, cryoablative, and cryopexy procedures in vitrectomy surgery. However, the probe had to be held within 1 mm of the retina to produce a discrete burn, since the light was transmitted by multiple parallel fibers resulting in a highly divergent beam. The probe also malfunctioned when it was not immersed in fluid to dissipate the heat generated.

In 1981, an improved source and delivery system for endophotocoagulation became available. Independently, Peyman and colleagues and Fleischman and colleagues described the delivery of argon laser energy through a quartz fiberoptic cable attached to a cannula that could be inserted into the human eye.[2,3] Advantages included a greater working distance from the retina, minimal heat production, and feasibility of using the device in gas-filled as well as in fluid-filled eyes. This subsequently became the standard for intraoperative laser therapy.

Other laser sources, including krypton and semiconductor diode lasers, have powered endolaser probes.[4] These light sources, especially the semiconductor diode, produce deeper retinal burns that may increase the risk of breaks in Bruch's membrane.

INDICATIONS

Endolaser photocoagulation has become a common procedure during vitrectomy surgery. It is indicated intraoperatively for panretinal photocoagulation of ischemic retina with neovascularization in diabetes mellitus, sickle cell disease, Eale's disease, and branch retinal vein occlusion.[5]

Endophotocoagulation also is valuable in repairing retinal detachments. Peripheral tears can be surrounded by several rows of burns. With giant retinal tears or proliferative vitreoretinopathy, multiple rows of endolaser spots delivered to the retina overlying the scleral buckle and around the tear may increase adherence of the retina to the retinal pigment epithelium. The endolaser has successfully cauterized subretinal neovascularization after evacuation of a subretinal hematoma through a retinotomy.[6] It also has functioned externally to perforate the choroid and drain subretinal fluid through a sclerotomy site.[7]

Additionally, the endolaser may prove valuable in nonretinal procedures, such as photoablation of the ciliary body in uncontrolled glaucoma.[8] Argon endolasers are currently being examined to produce full-thickness, ab interno sclerostomies. This technique may reduce the failure rate of filtering procedures in patients with neovascular glaucoma, aphakic or pseudophakic glaucoma, or previously failed trabeculectomies.[9] An endolaser probe recently has been modified to perform dacryocystorhinostomies.[10] Other indications may be expected in the future.

LASER TREATMENT

Optics

Viewing the fundus in a fluid-filled phakic eye through the operating microscope is accomplished with a planoconvex lens or a prism. A Landers lens (-95 D concave–convex lens) allows observation of a large retinal area while laser is applied. This causes minification of the fundus, and stereopsis is decreased, but the lens is useful to treat large areas quickly if the probe is kept a safe distance away from the retina (at least 3 mm). A Landers lens also offsets the induced high myopia in an air-filled phakic eye. Sometimes, no contact lens is necessary in a gas-filled aphakic eye. In an aphakic eye, laser may be performed on the peripheral retina indented into view. However, it is important to realize that the retina is closer to the probe with indentation. The laser power, duration setting, and the distance from the probe to the retina should be adjusted accordingly.

There usually is a water-cooled or air-cooled portable argon source in the operating suite, although in a few institutions, a fiberoptic guide from a remote source delivers the laser light to the operating suite and couples to the endolaser fiberoptic probe. An attenuated aiming beam of approximately 50 mW as well as light from the endoilluminator guide facilitate placement of laser burns. When the foot pedal is depressed, the safety shutter on the operating microscope is activated. After the filter rotates into place, a secondary switch closes and allows a preset full power beam to exit and photocoagulate the retina. In contrast to the slit-lamp delivery systems where the smallest image size is obtained by producing a convergent beam with the highest irradiance at the focal point, the beam at the tip of the endolaser probe is divergent. Therefore, the spot size is proportional to the distance between the endoprobe tip and the retinal surface. Divergence is affected also by the type of fiberoptic and the intraocular media. Since larger retinal areas are photocoagulated by increasing the endoprobe distance from the retina, more energy is needed to achieve the same burn intensity. This can be achieved by either increasing the power or increasing the duration.

Recently, diode semiconductor lasers have been developed with less wavelength scatter and less absorption by the lens and blood for ocular endophotocoagulation and slit-lamp delivery systems. Other advantages of diode lasers include a portable compact size, the ability to use standard electrical outlets, and simple air-cooling. Diode lasers currently available emit at approximately 810 nm, which is in the near infrared range of the spectrum. Since the sclera does not absorb this wavelength, cycloablation and retinal ablation can be done with external probes, similar to cryoablation or diathermy. Although this wavelength penetrates the ocular media well, only 18 percent of the light is absorbed by the retinal pigment epithelium, and 40 percent is absorbed by the choroid.[11] Deep penetration occurs, and care must be taken to prevent ruptures of Bruch's membrane. The power output in early diode laser models is limited. Longer exposures are required to create lesions comparable to those obtained with argon photocoagulation.[11]

More clinical studies are necessary to better define the efficiency of the diode laser in eye surgery. Because of the theoretical ease in constructing diode lasers, costs should decrease as the technology develops. There are prototypes of tunable diode lasers in the blue-green range.

Endolaser Operation

After operating suite personnel are wearing appropriate laser safety glasses, the laser is turned on and set on the standby mode. At this time, the physician should again check that there is a safety shutter in place to protect his eyes as well as the assistant's eyes. The laser parameters are turned to the lowest possible settings, usually 200 mW at 0.2 sec. Then the appropriate caliber endolaser probe (usually 19 or 20 gauge) and endoilluminator are inserted into the eye through pars plana ports. The laser is activated, and power as well as exposure duration are titrated until the desired lesion is achieved. A common mistake for the beginning surgeon is to maintain a constant power level as the eye is rotated toward the thin peripheral retina near the pars plana. This is especially true when the laser is applied near the endoprobe's entry site. A good clue that an adjustment should be made is that the burns become progressively whiter. If an inadvertent rupture of Bruch's membrane occurs during the endolaser procedure, the intraocular pressure should be increased by raising the infusion bottle height to stop the bleeding. Then two or three confluent rows of endolaser photocoagulation with either a large beam size or attenuated power should be delivered around the ruptured site. The inner retina within the arcades also may be damaged secondarily by intraretinal edema produced by argon blue-green energy.[5] This is avoided by using green wavelength argon and minimizing the amount of coagulation within the arcades.

A few retina specialists perform peripheral endolaser using an indirect ophthalmoscope rather than an operating microscope. Safety goggles are worn, or appropriate blocking filters are placed in the oculars of the indirect ophthalmoscope.[12] Relying on eyelid closure without filters at the time of discharge is extremely dangerous. With the aiming beam at its highest setting, the surgeon can see a dim spot at the point of retinal irradiance while wearing the safety goggles. Using indirect ophthalmoscopic guidance, the endolaser is moved to appropriate locations, and photocoagulation is administered. This procedure is very difficult. The image is inverted, so landmarks must be well known to determine if the probe is moving in the intended direction. Second, the image is minified, with stereopsis markedly decreased. Retinal tears can be created easily by misguiding the endoprobe as well as by misjudging the distance between the probe and the retina. Laser treatment of the peripheral retina in the operating suite is safer using the binocular indirect ophthalmoscope laser delivery system.

Clinical use of the diode laser endoprobe is similar to the argon probe. However, since infrared light is being used, a fixed far red–infrared filter is in place, which gives the retina a slight bluish tinge but does not otherwise interfere with the view. The probe has to be held slightly closer, and usually longer exposures are needed. As a general rule, the surgeon should change duration concurrently with power so that if 0.1 W and 0.1 sec are not sufficient, 0.2 W and 0.2 sec are tried, and successively higher wattage as well as duration exposures are used. Some patients with highly pigmented retinal pigment epithelium and choroid require shorter durations and exposure times to get adequate burns. Patients with moderate pigmentation may require up to 0.6 W and 0.6 sec, and in lightly pigmented eyes, especially with air in the vitreous cavity, higher powers and longer duration times are necessary.

Troubleshooting

If the endolaser probe is not functioning, several things should be examined. (1) Obviously, the laser power source must be turned on and functioning. (2) Connections may become loose. (3) The fiberoptics to the endoprobe may become damaged. This is especially true if they have been crushed, twisted, or reused multiple times. (4) Intraoperatively, small air bubbles can be produced at the tip of the endolaser probe. These air bubbles will greatly attenuate the beam. The endolaser probe may appear to have decreased efficiency or not function. If the laser power is increased and the bubbles dislodge, a Bruch's membrane rupture may occur. Therefore, if the endoprobe ceases to function intraoperatively, the endoilluminator should be touched to the tip of the endolaser probe to dislodge any bubbles. (5) Repeated discharges fired too rapidly will overheat the laser, causing locking of the safety filter. This is more likely to occur in air-cooled lasers. Allow the laser to cool in standby mode for a few minutes before resuming.

REFERENCES

1. Charles S: Endophotocoagulation. *Ophthalmol Times* 1979;4:68–69.
2. Peyman GA, Grisolano JM, Palacio MN: Intraocular photocoagulation with the argon-krypton laser. *Arch Ophthalmol* 1980;98:2062–2064.
3. Fleischman JA, Swartz M, Dixon JA: Argon laser endophotocoagulation: an intraoperative trans-pars plana technique. *Arch Ophthalmol* 1981;99:1610–1612.
4. Duker JS, Federman JL, Schubert H, Talbot C: Semiconductor diode laser endophotocoagulation. *Ophthalmic Surg* 1989;20:717–719.
5. Acheson RW, Capon M, Cooling RJ, Leaver PK, Marshall J, McLeod D: Intraocular argon laser photocoagulation. *Eye* 1987;1:97–105.
6. Thomas MA, Halperin LS: Subretinal endolaser treatment of a choroidal bleeding site. *Am J Ophthalmol* 1990;109:742–744.
7. Bovino JA, Marcus DF, Nelsen PT: Argon laser choroidotomy for drainage of subretinal fluid. *Arch Ophthalmol* 1985;103:443–444.
8. Zarbin MA, Michels RG, de Bustros S, Quigley HA, Patel A: Endolaser treatment of the ciliary body for severe glaucoma. *Ophthalmology* 1988;95:1639–1648.
9. Jaffe GJ, Mieler WF, Radius RL, Kincaid MC, Massaro BM, Abrams GW: Ab interno sclerostomy with a high-powered argon endolaser: clinicopathologic correlation. *Arch Ophthalmol* 1989;107:1183–1185.
10. Massaro BM, Gonnering RS, Harris GJ: Endonasal laser dacryocystorhinostomy: a new approach to nasolacrimal duct obstruction. *Arch Ophthalmol* 1990;108:1172–1176.
11. Puliafito CA, Deutsch TF, Boll J, To K: Semiconductor laser endophotocoagulation of the retina. *Arch Ophthalmol* 1987;105:424–427.
12. Grisolano J, Peyman GA: An automatic laser filter for the indirect ophthalmoscope. *Retina* 1987;7:32–33.

CHAPTER 17

Binocular Indirect Ophthalmoscope Laser Photocoagulator

Jose S. Pulido and Karen M. Joos

- ■ **Introduction**
- ■ **Indications**
- ■ **Laser Treatment**
  - **Optics**
  - **Technique**
  - **Troubleshooting**
- ■ **References**

INTRODUCTION

Mizuno originally described the use of an argon blue-green laser photocoagulation system coupled to a binocular indirect ophthalmoscope in 1981.[1] The laser modified for interchangeable indirect ophthalmoscope or slit-lamp delivery was used successfully in patients with diabetic retinopathy, vein occlusions, retinal detachments, and retinopathy of prematurity.[2,3] The binocular indirect ophthalmoscope laser photocoagulator (BIOLP) has been refined recently to include a better filter system and argon green energy capability.[4]

The fiberoptic carrying the laser beam is attached to an indirect ophthalmoscope. Depressing the laser pedal activates a mechanical shutter to flip a barrier filter into place to protect the surgeon's eyes at the time of discharge. A different system uses a fixed barrier filter with a coaxial He-Ne aiming beam to guide delivery. A handheld 20 or 30 D condensing lens focuses the laser and allows viewing of the fundus through the indirect ophthalmoscope. Newer BIOLPs also deliver krypton red with an appropriate filter. This permits treatment through nuclear sclerotic cataracts and mild hemorrhages. BIOLPs also can deliver near infrared light from diode lasers. This system has fixed infrared filters in place, obviating heavy shutter systems on the binocular indirect ophthalmoscope.

INDICATIONS

The BIOLP is especially useful for treating people who cannot sit at the slit lamp, for example, invalids and children. Since a contact lens is not necessary with the BIOLP, this method is safer in eyes with recently sutured lacerations and may be less frightening than the slit-lamp laser delivery system (Table 17–1). It can be used also in the operating room with sedation or general anesthesia in uncooperative patients. The BIOLP is valuable for panretinal or focal photocoagulation of the peripheral retina (Table 17–2). Since its accuracy is about 200 μm, the macular region probably should be avoided.

Individual peripheral tears can be treated completely without the use of cryopexy. If necessary, scleral depression can be performed to visualize the peripheral retina. Depression will mechanically approximate the retinal pigment epithelium to the retina and permit photoretinopexy when some subretinal fluid remains after retinal reattachment procedures. Even eyes after partial gas exchanges or pneumatic retinopexy procedures can be manipulated to displace the bubble for laser retinopexy.[5] It also may be helpful in retinal reattachment surgery when the hole is not identified. Photocoagulation over large areas of the retina produces less blood–retinal barrier breakdown than obtained with cryopexy.[6]

LASER TREATMENT

Optics

As with any other delivery system, the energy delivered to an area of the retina is dependent on the power and duration of exposure and inversely proportional to the spot size. As opposed to a slit-lamp delivery system where the distance between the patient and the slit lamp is fixed, there is no fixed position of either the patient, the lens, or the ophthalmologist in the BIOLP system. Therefore, spot size variation is more common, and Bruch's membrane ruptures may occur. Thus, stability of the operator and patient is important. By bringing the operator closer to the patient, the retinal image will appear magnified, and the laser beam usually will subtend a smaller part of the ret-

TABLE 17–1. COMPARISONS BETWEEN BINOCULAR INDIRECT OPHTHALMOSCOPE LASER PHOTOCOAGULATOR (BIOLP) AND SLIT-LAMP LASER DELIVERY SYSTEMS FOR RETINAL PHOTOCOAGULATION

BIOLP	Slit-Lamp Delivery system
1. Noncontact	1. Contact lens required
2. Easy to use with patient in a supine position for invalids	2. Slit-lamp positioning of the patient is important
3. Spot size is difficult to control well	3. Spot size is better controlled
4. Aiming accuracy is about 200 μm (not for macular use)	4. Reliable aiming accuracy
5. Variable power with change in head position of the operator or patient (easier to rupture Bruch's membrane)	5. Less power delivery variability
6. Light scattered back to the operator's eyes	6. Less scatter of light to the operator
7. Head and neck fatigue from weight of laser attachments to the indirect ophthalmoscope	7. Less operator fatigue
8 Ora and far periphery easily treated with scleral indentation	8. Difficult to treat the far periphery and ora serrata
9. Patient's head can be manipulated to treat around gas bubbles	9. Difficult to treat around gas bubbles

TABLE 17–2. INDICATIONS FOR BINOCULAR INDIRECT OPHTHALMOSCOPE LASER PHOTOCOAGULATION

Peripheral scatter or focal: Adults/children
    Sickle cell retinopathy
    Proliferative diabetic retinopathy
    Venous occlusive disease
    Retinopathy of prematurity
    Incontinentia pigmenti
    Coats' disease
    von Hippel angiomas
    Near the ora with scleral depression
Retinal detachment
    Wall-off
    Pneumatic laser retinopexy
    External choroidotomies

ina, resulting in a smaller burn size. Conversely, increasing the distance between the patient and the operator will minify the image and usually cause enlargement of the laser spot size on the retina.

Besides the position of the patient, condensing lens, and operator, variables, including focal length of the laser cone, condensing lens power, and the refractive power of the patient's eye, will affect the retinal burn size. Spot size variations of the laser are achieved by adjusting a zoom telescope in some systems or exchanging a fixed lens in other systems. This changes the focal point of the beam. Micron spot size indicators are placed on some BIOLPs, but these are only rough estimations. Correlation of the aiming beam size with retinal vessel and disc size should be made before extensive use.

Spot size on the retina can be varied by changing the power of the condensing lens. Just as the size of the retinal image in space can be altered by changing condensing lenses, an external beam of light can subtend a larger or smaller area on the retina. The relationship is an inverse one. With more magnification of the retina, the beam of light subtends a smaller area of the total retina and is minified. Conversely, with less magnification of the retinal image, the beam of light subtends a larger area in the retina, and, therefore, the laser spot size is larger. In a 60 D model eye, a 20 D condensing lens will produce a retinal image with three times magnification (60 D divided by 20 D = 3×), whereas an external coherent laser beam will be minified to one third at the retinal surface. A 10 D lens will cause more magnification of the retinal image (60 D divided by 10 D = 6×) and, therefore, more minification of the laser spot size (1/6 of the original size) on the retina because a coherent light will illuminate a smaller retinal area. A 30 D lens will cause less magnification of the retinal image (60 D divided by 30 D = 2×) and, therefore, less minification of the retinal laser burn (1/2 of the original size).

In a myopic eye, the dioptric power of the eye is greater than the 60 D model eye. Therefore, more magnification of the retinal image and more minification of the retinal laser beam spot size occur. For example, in a −20 D eye, using a 20 D condensing lens, the magnification of the image is 80 D divided by 20 D = 4×, as opposed to 3× in a model eye of 60 D. Minification of the retinal laser spot size is one fourth, as opposed to one third of the original spot size for the emmetropic model eye. Therefore, the change is a 25 percent reduction in spot size (three fourths = 75 percent of the spot size in an emmetropic eye). In a hyperopic eye, the power is less than in the emmetropic 60 D model eye. Therefore, less magnification of the retinal image and less minification of the external laser beam spot occur. For example, using a 20 D condensing lens to treat a +20 D hyperopic eye will produce a retinal image of 40 divided by 20 = 2× magnification, in comparison to the 60 D divided by 20 D = 3× magnification for a model emmetropic eye. Minification in a hyperopic eye is less than that in an emmetropic eye. The burn size will be (approximately 50%) 1.5× larger than laser spots in the model emmetropic eye. A gas-filled phakic eye is similar to the highly myopic system, and an aphakic eye is similar to the hyperopic system.

Technique

Appropriate safety goggles are to be worn by ancillary personnel. Topical 0.5 percent proparacaine hydrochloride is applied to the patient's eye. The patient is placed supine or comfortably upright against a headrest.

The BIOLP functions as an indirect ophthalmoscope with fiberoptic illumination that is adjustable by a rheostat on the light source. An additional fiberoptic cable connects the indirect ophthalmoscope to the laser source. Aiming beam intensity, treatment power, and treatment duration controls are located on the laser console. Initially, a low power setting of 200 mW and pulse duration of 0.1 to 0.2 sec are used. The indirect may have an attenuated argon aiming beam with a mobile safety filter that moves into place before release of the laser beam after the foot pedal is pressed or may have an aiming beam from a He-Ne source with a fixed argon safety filter. With the aiming beam on and the laser set on standby, the retina can be scanned to become comfortable with the view. Then the retinal burn size can be adjusted by turning a zoom lens mounted on the indirect ophthalmoscope or by changing a fixed lens on the indirect ophthalmoscope in other systems. A 28 D or 30 D condensing lens will increase the size of the retinal burn in comparison to a 20 D lens.[7] Power and burn duration are adjusted for the amount of fundus pigmentation and media opacity.

Troubleshooting

The size of the laser spot is dependent on multiple factors, including patient position, lens power, and position of the ophthalmologist. Lens aberrations may affect burn size and produce oval-shaped burns in the periphery. A clear view of the targeted area of retina is required before firing. Additionally, the laser power must be reduced during scleral indentation. If a rupture of Bruch's membrane occurs with hemorrhage, pressure should be applied to the globe, followed by three rows of laser burns with attenuated power around the break.[7]

With the BIOLP in a darkened room, the retina and not the whole eye is viewed. Laser energy can be applied accidentally to the cornea during repositioning movements and not be noted until the retinal view becomes cloudy.[8] Therefore, it is important to use low power settings, avoid short duration bursts, obtain the clearest image of the retina with the aiming beam as round and clear as possible, and examine the quality of retinal burns being produced. If poor quality retinal burns are produced with adequate power settings, adjust the positioning of the patient and make sure a yellow-tinted condensing lens is not being used, since it will reduce the amount of light that reaches the retina. Also, examine the patient's cornea and lens for evidence of inadvertent photocoagulation. If the machine is calibrated to argon blue-green and argon green only is used, it is important to remember that the power actually is less than indicated. Finally, peripheral glare generated during retinal ablation can be minimized by wearing dark clothing while operating the machine.

REFERENCES

1. Mizuno K: Binocular indirect argon laser photocoagulator. *Br J Ophthalmol* 1981; 65:425–428.
2. Mizuno K, Takaku Y: Dual delivery system for argon laser photocoagulation: improved techniques of the binocular indirect argon laser photocoagulator. *Arch Ophthalmol* 1983;101:648–652.
3. Friberg TR: Clinical experience with a binocular indirect ophthalmoscope laser deliver system. *Retina* 1987;7:28–31.
4. Whitacre MM, Manoukian N, Mainster MA: Argon indirect ophthalmoscopic photocoagulation: reduced potential phototoxicity with a fixed safety filter. *Br J Ophthalmol* 1990;74:233–234.
5. Friberg TR, Eller AW: Pneumatic repair of primary and secondary retinal detachments using a binocular indirect ophthalmoscope laser delivery system. *Ophthalmology* 1988;95:187–193.
6. Jaccoma EH, Conway BP, Campochiaro PA: Cryotherapy causes extensive breakdown of the blood retinal barrier: a comparison with argon laser photocoagulation. *Arch Ophthalmol* 1985;103:1728–1730.
7. Friberg TR: Principles of photocoagulation using binocular indirect ophthalmoscope laser delivery systems. *Int Ophthalmol Clin* 1990;30:89–94.
8. Rubinfeld RS, Pilkerton AR, Zimmerman LE: A corneal complication of indirect ophthalmic laser delivery systems. *Am J Ophthalmol* 1990;110:206–208.

CHAPTER 18

Complications of Laser Photocoagulation

Peter R. Pavan, E. George Rosanelli, Deen G. King, and Thomas A. Weingeist

INTRODUCTION

Many complications of argon laser retinal photocoagulation, iridotomy, and trabeculoplasty can be minimized or avoided through proper technique. Other undesired effects often resolve without permanent sequelae if properly managed.

ARGON LASER PANRETINAL PHOTOCOAGULATION

The complications of argon panretinal photocoagulation (APRP) can be divided conveniently into four categories: transient changes, mild, unavoidable side effects, potentially severe but avoidable complications, and severe, unavoidable, adverse results.

TRANSIENT CHANGES

Many transient changes after APRP occur only when a large area of the retina is treated in one session or in closely spaced sessions. These changes are due to the exudation of fluid from the choroid and retina and can be alarming to the novice photocoagulator. Fortunately, most are easily managed and resolve without affecting the final visual outcome.

After the equivalent of 800 or more spots of the 500 μm size, peripheral choroidal detachments may develop. The exudation of fluid into the posterior segment can induce a myopic shift in the patient's refractive error by causing a forward displacement of the lens–iris diaphragm. Uncorrected, this myopic shift can reduce visual acuity dramatically. Both patient and physician are reassured when placing minus sphere over the prelaser correction restores good vision. Postlaser choroidal detachments and myopic shift usually occur within 1 day of laser therapy and spontaneously resolve without sequelae within days to weeks.[1,2]

The forward movement of the lens–iris diaphragm often is associated with a rise in the intraocular pressure. The pressure probably rises because exudation of fluid into the posterior segment occurs faster than aqueous can leave the anterior chamber through the trabecular meshwork. Pressure elevations have been recorded as early as 10 minutes after APRP and can reach 50 to 60 mm Hg within a few hours as the anterior chamber continues to shallow. A significant number of eyes will go on to close the angle. The open-angle and closed-angle pressure elevation seen in the hours to days after extensive APRP usually does not require therapy because the pressure elevation is only moderate. However, should the pressure reach 50 mm Hg or more within the first few hours of laser therapy with either an open or closed angle, treatment is indicated. Dilation with cycloplegics deepens the anterior chamber and prevents pupillary block. Timolol and acetazolamide (Diamox) lessen fluid flow into the eye from the ciliary body, decreasing intraocular pressure. These measures can be stopped after a few days.[3]

Exudation of fluid under the retina causes neurosensory detachments. In the periphery, these can assume a rhegmatogenous configuration reaching the ora serrata. Atrophic retinal holes may develop in the detachment in the center of the recently placed retinal burns. Obviously, the combination of a rhegmatogenous-appearing detachment associated with retinal holes is a worrisome finding. Although they do not have shifting subretinal fluid, the spontaneous resolution of these detachments within 1 to 2 weeks shows that they are really exudative rather than rhegmatogenous in nature.[1,4,5]

Neurosensory detachments can occur also in the posterior pole. When the fovea is involved, the visual decrease can be profound and is uncorrectable with lenses. As in the periphery, the neurosensory detachment resolves within a few weeks. Vision continues to improve after the detachment is no longer detectable, taking as long as a few months to reach prelaser levels.[5]

Finally, the exudation of fluid within the retina can cause cystoid macular edema. Although it usually regresses, cystoid edema may lead to a lasting decrease in acuity.[6]

Most of the changes secondary to exudation of fluid can be avoided by giving APRP in divided sittings. Each session should have no more than 400 to 600 of the 500 μm size spots, with the intensity of each spot just enough to cause definite retinal whitening. Treating preexisting macular edema by focal photocoagulation before initiating scatter therapy may decrease the risk of visual loss.[7] However, eyes with advanced neovascularization of the anterior segment, patients commuting from long distances, and advanced posterior segment neovascularization with early vitreous hemorrhage are situations where many experts feel APRP should be completed in one session. Fortunately, the final visual outcome is the same whether APRP is given in one dose or divided doses.[4]

Two other transient changes are seen after APRP. If the Rodenstock lens is used, air can come between the lens and the cornea without being visible to the surgeon. When this happens, the corneal epithelium is coagulated. The white, opaque, coagulated epithelium is replaced by normal epithelial cells within 1 day. Occasionally, a laser burn will hit a retinal vessel. As long as the spot is larger than the vessel diameter and the intensity is just enough to obtain definite retinal whitening, the worst that will happen is temporary vascular spasm. If a small, hot spot size is used, a hole can be punched in the vessel wall, resulting in massive, uncontrollable, intraocular bleeding.

MILD, UNAVOIDABLE SIDE EFFECTS

Mild decreases may occur in four visual functions after APRP. First, damage to the short ciliary nerves as they course through the choroid causes a partial internal ophthalmoplegia. This results in a larger, poorly reactive pupil and in a decrease in accommodation. Latent hyperopes and patients in the fourth and fifth decades may need reading glasses or bifocals for the first time after APRP. Patients who already use bifocals may require an increase in their add. There is no way to avoid the majority of the 6 to 10 short ciliary nerves during APRP because most cannot be seen.[8–10]

Peripheral field loss also occurs after APRP. If 500 μm spots are used and ½ to 1 spot of untreated retina is left between laser spots as recommended in the Diabetic Retinopathy Study protocol, adequate therapy can be given while leaving the patient with functional peripheral vision.[11] Some clinicians will place new laser spots between old laser burns if the new vessels do not go away or continue to proliferate after a routine, complete APRP. Such retreatment often leaves the patient with tunnel vision, a severe visual handicap. Furthermore, if the macula later develops a traction detachment, severe edema, or severe ischemia, the eye has no useful vision. Additional 500 μm spots in the far periphery or one to two rows of 200 μm spots within the arcades rarely cause visual problems and are preferable to adding new spots between old burns. Once complete APRP and this extra laser therapy have been given, techniques other than APRP, such as peripheral cryopexy or vitrectomy, should be considered if progression of the proliferative retinopathy causes, or has an overwhelming likelihood of causing, severe visual loss.

Central vision also can be decreased by APRP. Using complicated statistical methods, the Diabetic Retinopathy Study showed that APRP causes a decrease of 1 line in 11 percent of eyes and a decrease equal to or greater than 2 lines in 3 percent of eyes.[11] The reason for this central vision loss is unknown. Of course, in any one eye, it is usually impossible to tell if a decrease in vision after APRP is due to the treatment or to progression of the diabetic retinopathy.

Finally, the already decreased scotopic vision of eyes with proliferative diabetic retinopathy is further impaired. Although formal tests show that the rod-cone break is only delayed an additional 1.2 minutes and the final rod threshold is only elevated an additional 0.4 log units, these differences are noted by a surprising number of patients.[12]

It is important to warn patients of these four visual changes induced by APRP. Most will accept these costs when the need for laser therapy to decrease their chance of severe visual loss is explained. Despite the presence of high-risk characteristics, some may elect to delay laser treatment once these potential side effects are enumerated. An example is the interstate trucker with 20/40 visual acuity in his better eye. A further decrease in central acuity would result in revocation of his license and loss of employment. The decision to treat or not to treat should always be left to the informed patient.

POTENTIALLY SEVERE BUT AVOIDABLE COMPLICATIONS

The most dreaded complication of APRP is accidental photocoagulation of the fovea. This catastrophe usually happens in one of five ways. Most commonly, physicians photocoagulate the macula because they think they are treating the peripheral retina with one of the mirrors of a Goldmann lens when, in reality, the aiming beam has slipped into the center of the lens, and they are looking directly at the posterior pole. The probability of this error can be lessened by using the Pavan Rotation Test. If the aiming beam is reflecting off a mirror, rotation of the lens will cause the aiming beam to move grossly in relation to retinal landmarks. However, if the aiming beam is going directly through the center of the lens without bouncing off a mirror, rotation of the lens will cause little or no movement of the spot on the retina (Fig. 18–1). By always performing this simple test when using the mirrors of a Goldmann, or similar, lens, the photocoagulator can be assured that the aiming beam is, indeed, hitting a mirror.

The laser beam can move into the fovea when the photocoagulator is not looking into the eye. This mishap usually happens when the physician momentarily diverts the gaze to flip the safety switch or to adjust the power. To avoid this error, the control box should be positioned so the photocoagulator can turn the safety switch on and off without gazing away from the fundus. To adjust power, the laser is turned off by feeling the safety switch, power is varied while looking at the dial, retinal landmarks are then rechecked, and the laser is turned back on by flipping the safety switch while the photocoagulator continues to gaze at the fundus. Alternatively, the laser can be adjusted by an assistant seated by the controls.

The fovea also can be photocoagulated accidentally when using the centermost part of the steepest (and biggest) mirror of the Goldmann lens. This part of the mirror directs burns more posteriorly. It is possible to reach the fovea, especially from the temporal side, in aphakic patients by having the patient look toward the mirror or by tilting the mirror toward the center of the cornea. The newly designed Karickhoff lens has an even steeper mirror, which can easily direct burns into the fovea. To prevent accidental irradiation of the fovea with the mirror, a few rows of barrier burns are placed first temporal to the macula using the center of the Goldmann lens or a nonmirrored contact lens with a plano anterior surface (Fig. 18–2). The physician then makes sure not to treat posterior to these barrier burns when using a mirror. When APRP is done in divided sessions, barrier burns should be placed only in the quadrant, third, or half of the retina to be treated that day. If all the barrier burns are placed at the first sitting but the periphery is treated in divided sessions 1 week apart, the barrier burns may be hard to see during the second and third sessions because their acute retinal whiteness has faded and chorioretinal scarring has not yet fully developed.

The fovea can be hit when the patient flinches unexpectedly. Usually, the patient attempts to close both eyes. The resulting Bell's phenomenon rotates the fovea under the aiming beam if burns are being given inferior to the macula. APRP is best initiated nasal to the disc. If the patient repeatedly flinches, a retrobulbar injection before treating under the macula will lessen the danger of a foveal burn.

Finally, the Rodenstock lens often is touted for the panoramic view it gives the photocoagulator. This enables one to always know where treatment

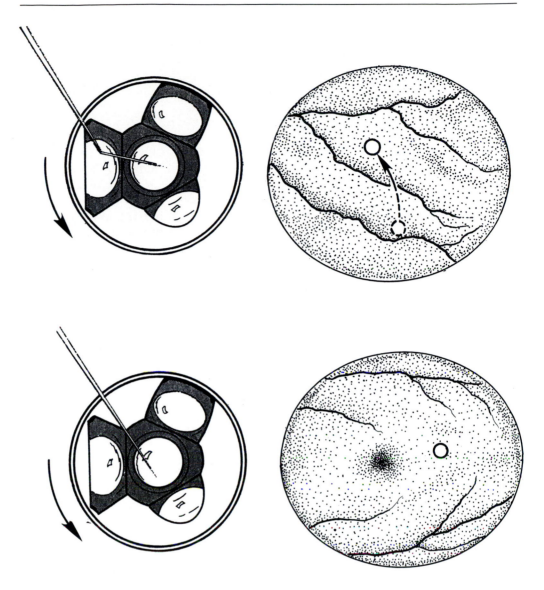

Figure 18–1. When the aiming beam is reflected off a mirror, rotation of the lens causes gross movement of the aiming spot on the retina. When the aiming beam goes directly through the central part of the lens, rotation causes little or no movement of the spot on the retina.

is being given in relationship to the macula. However, at least one retinal specialist has accidentally hit the fovea when momentarily forgetting that the Rodenstock lens gives an inverted, reversed image of the retina.

In addition to shunning the fovea, the physician should never treat preretinal or vitreous membranes. Heating preretinal membranes with laser light causes their contraction and may lead to detachment of the underlying retina. Direct treatment of vitreous membranes also causes their contraction and may result in detachment of the retinal areas to which they are adherent.

Hot, short spots are also to be eschewed. As previously mentioned, this type of spot can perforate a vessel, causing massive intraocular hemorrhage. More commonly, hot, short spots rupture Bruch's membrane. This rupture is seen as a punched-out, depigmented area without overlying whitening of the

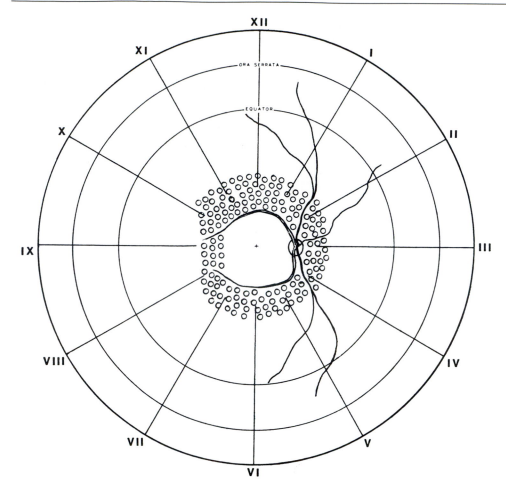

Figure 18–2. Barrier burns have been placed around the macula, using the center of the Goldmann lens or a nonmirrored contact lens with a plano anterior surface. When the mirror is used to place burns in the periphery, care is taken never to photocoagulate posterior to the barrier burns.

retina and is associated commonly with a choroidal, subretinal, or vitreous hemorrhage. Although the hemorrhage usually is self-contained, it is best to apply pressure to the globe through the contact lens and to treat the source of bleeding with larger, hotter, longer duration spots until the blood stops oozing. A late complication of rupture of Bruch's membrane is the occurrence of subretinal neovascular membranes or the growth of vessels from the choroid into the vitreous. Subretinal new vessels may be eradicated successfully with laser, but choroidovitreal neovascular ingrowth is unresponsive to any treatment and has a poor prognosis.[13,14]

Hot spots are commonly made in one of four ways. First, the photocoagulator may accommodate, causing the laser beam to be out of focus on the retina when the retina is in focus for the operator's eyes. To get retinal whitening with the diffuse laser beam, the power will be turned up. When the photocoagulator then relaxes the accommodation, the laser beam will come into sharp focus, and overcoagulation will occur. To prevent this accident, the photocoagulator should try pulling back on the joystick to make the aiming beam spot as small as possible on the retina and fire again before increasing the power to achieve a retinal burn. Second, less power is needed to photocoagulate thinner peripheral retina with a mirror than to treat thicker posterior retina through the center of a Goldmann-type lens. Hence, when changing from the center to the mirror, the power must be adjusted down, or excessively intense burns will be given. Third, hot spots occur when treating a fundus through variable media opacities. The power is turned up when trying to penetrate through a dense media opacity. When the laser beam then moves to an area with a less dense media opacity, the power must be reduced to avoid overcoagulation. Finally, hot burns occur if the power is not turned down when going from edematous to nonedematous retina.

Although accidental treatment of the fovea and choroidovitreal neovascular ingrowth are the most dreaded complications of APRP, they are, fortunately, rare. By far the most common error for the novice photocoagulator is the administration of inadequate APRP. Large areas may be left untreated due to difficulties with patient cooperation. A retrobulbar injection frequently makes the treatment easier by lessening any pain associated with the laser and by decreasing the patient's perception of the bright lights from the slit lamp and laser. Lidocaine 2 percent without epinephrine or hyaluronidase usually is sufficient.

An orbital hemorrhage after retrobulbar lidocaine can cause occlusion of the central retinal artery. Despite excellent primate research, which suggests that the retina can do without its intrinsic blood supply for up to 90 minutes with full recovery of function, all central retinal artery occlusions secondary to retrobulbar hemorrhage should be treated promptly.[15] Human retinas with diabetic retinopathy may not have the same endurance for prolonged ischemia that the healthy monkey retina has in the experimental situation. If a canthotomy fails to reestablish flow in the central retinal artery, an inferior cantholysis should be done immediately (Fig. 18–3). Cantholysis has always reestablished flow in the authors' experience. The APRP can then be given.

The akinesis induced by retrobulbar injection frequently causes problems in viewing the area of retina between that easily seen through the central portion of the contact lens and that easily visualized through the steepest, largest mirror of the Goldmann lens. This can result in a ring of unlasered retina around the posterior pole (Fig. 18–4). This ring can be treated in one of three ways. First, proper manipulation of the plano contact lens and a Goldmann three-mirror lens will allow treatment of this difficult area. The posterior part

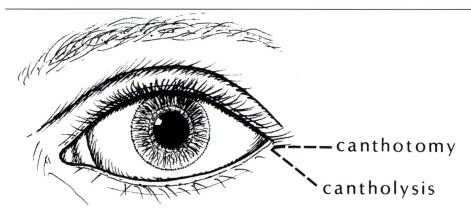

Figure 18–3. Lateral canthotomy may not relieve orbital tension adequately in the presence of a retrobulbar hemorrhage. An inferior cantholysis creates significantly more room in the orbit. A lateral canthotomy is performed by making a horizontal cut through all of the tissues at the lateral canthus, including the conjunctiva. The lateral canthal commissure should be clamped for 1 minute with a hemostat before cutting the tissue with a scissors. An inferior cantholysis is created by directing the scissors inferotemporally and severing the inferior crus of the lateral canthal tendon without further skin cuts.

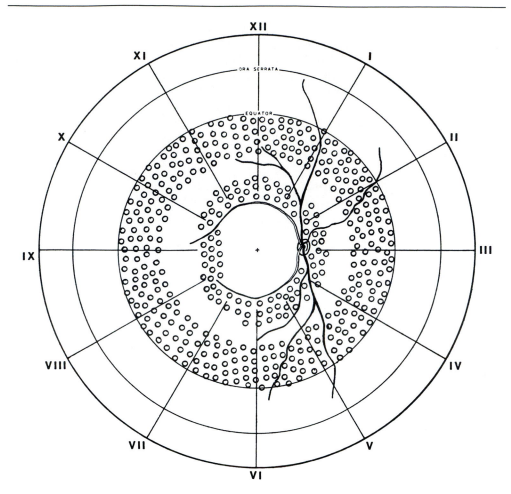

Figure 18–4. Ring of untreated retina around the posterior pole due to difficulties viewing this area with a Goldmann lens.

---

of the more horizontal meridians of the ring can be seen through a plano lens by swinging the slit lamp to one side and viewing obliquely. The vertical meridians are best seen by tilting the head and pressing slightly on the contact lens to move the eye up or down (Fig. 18–5). It is best to use a nonmirrored plano contact lens for these maneuvers. The mirrored Goldmann lens is bulky, and its excursions are limited by the orbital rim. The peripheral portion of the untreated ring can be lasered by tilting the largest Goldmann mirror toward the cornea while exerting pressure on the opposite limbus (Fig. 18–6). Alternatively, the steepest mirror of the Karickhoff lens or a Rodenstock lens can be used to apply APRP in the ring area.

Opacities of the lens or vitreous can result in inadequate therapy. Peripheral cortical spokes are best overcome by reducing the spot size to 200 μm and increasing the duration of the burns to 0.2 sec. This maneuver can also help when working through nuclear sclerosis or vitreous hemorrhage. However, if there is sufficient nuclear sclerosis, lenticular protein can be coagulated by laser, leaving a permanent opacity. Settings more intense than 200 μm, 0.2 sec, and 1.0 W should not be used. Krypton red penetrates nuclear sclerotic lenses and vitreous hemorrhage better than does argon blue-green.[16] If even krypton red cannot penetrate, panretinal cryopexy[17] or cataract extraction followed by laser treatment should be considered.

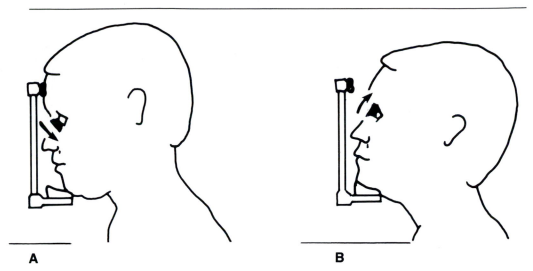

Figure 18–5. A. By tilting the head forward, placing the chin back as far as possible, and pressing on the nonmirrored contact lens with a plano anterior surface to push the eye down, more peripheral retina can be treated inferiorly. **B.** Maneuver is reversed to treat more peripherally superiorly.

SEVERE, UNAVOIDABLE, ADVERSE SIDE EFFECTS

Excessive fibrosis with contraction of preretinal and vitreous membranes after APRP can cause distortion of the macula and a drop in visual acuity. Whether this fibrosis is due to laser or is part of the natural history of diabetic retinopathy is not known. It can occur suddenly in eyes without laser treatment. However, if it happens just after APRP, the patient usually attributes the decrease in vision to laser treatment. Fortunately, this is not a common complication, and it is the only severe, unavoidable, adverse effect of APRP. It is best treated using vitrectomy techniques.

ARGON LASER MACULAR PHOTOCOAGULATION FOR MACULAR EDEMA

Macular edema caused by diabetes and branch retinal vein occlusion is usually treated without a retrobulbar anesthetic injection. As a consequence, treatment should never be started directly inferior to fixation. If the patient blinks when the first laser spot is administered, the point of fixation will rotate down into the path of the laser beam. Also avoid initiating treatment just below a major retinal vessel. If reflex blinking rotates the vessel into the laser beam, vascular spasm or occlusion could occur. Because small spot sizes are sometimes used in macular photocoagulation, perforation of the vessel wall could cause a vitreous hemorrhage. Only after acclimating the patient to the laser and gaining full cooperation should these high risk areas be treated.

Small, hot spots of short duration should be avoided in the macula. Since the results of the Early Treatment Diabetic Retinopathy Study were first published, two reports have documented the growth of subretinal neovascular membranes in 12 patients after focal argon photocoagulation for clinically significant macular edema. The authors concluded that this serious complication

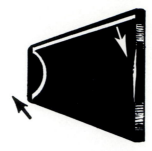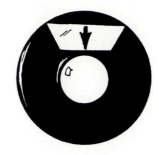

Figure 18–6. To view (and treat) more posteriorly using the large mirror of the Goldmann lens, tilt the lens toward the center of the cornea and exert pressure on the limbus opposite the mirror by pushing on the lens.

was related to the use of small-size, short-duration laser or intense laser burns or both. Should a hot spot be placed, careful follow-up with Amsler grid testing and fluorescein angiography may allow detection of subretinal new vessels at an early stage, improving the prognosis.[18,19]

Spread of laser burns toward fixation when working close to the center of the macula can occur with the argon blue-green laser secondary to absorption of the blue wavelengths by the xanthophyll. This undesirable effect can be avoided by using an attachment that removes the blue wavelength from the argon beam, leaving only green, or by using a yellow wavelength from another type of laser, such as a tunable dye laser. Green and yellow have the advantage of being well absorbed by blood, making photocoagulation of microaneurysms easier. Like green and yellow, krypton red and tunable dye red are not absorbed by the xanthophyll. However, red wavelengths usually are not used for diabetic macular edema because they are not absorbed well by hemoglobin.[20]

ARGON LASER IRIDOTOMY

The application of argon laser iridotomy for the treatment of narrow-angle glaucoma steadily increased to replace surgical iridectomy in the mid 1970s. The majority of published data are on continuous wave argon lasers, but pulsed argon lasers also have been used with similar success rates and complications.[21] The iridotomy may be accomplished using a thermal laser, such as the argon, or by photodisruption, such as in the case of the Nd:YAG laser. The relative ease of Nd:YAG iridotomies has caused a decline in the frequency of argon laser iridotomies, although the argon laser iridotomy offers some distinct advantages.

Argon laser photocoagulation is the preferred mode for the formation of an iridotomy in eyes that are prone to hemorrhage, such as in patients with neovascularization of the iris surface, in the presence of large iris vessels, or in patients with uveitis who have dilated iris blood vessels. The argon laser also allows the surgeon to modify the anterior chamber depth by applying large, low-power burns that will coagulate and stretch the superficial iris, thus deepening the chamber before application of full-power treatment to obtain perforation. This is a means of protecting the corneal endothelium and is a modality not available to those using a photodisruptor. Pretreatment of the iridotomy site using an argon laser for photocoagulation often is beneficial even when the photodisruptor is used to perforate the iris.

Nonperforation is the most commonly encountered complication of iridotomy. First, migration of fresh tissue into a site with each additional burn can result in a large, partial-thickness excoriation rather than a full-thickness hole. The chance of tissue migration can be minimized by preoperative stretching of the iris by a miotic (e.g., 1–2 percent pilocarpine). Short duration burns of 0.05 sec or less will produce less coagulation of surrounding tissue and lessen pigment migration when the problem is encountered.

The 12-o'clock position is least likely to induce monocular diplopia, but care must be taken to position the iridotomy site at a location that will not be occluded by bubbles and pigment liberated during the initial part of the treatment. Bubble formation can be minimized by employing a drilling technique, with the majority of the treatment directed deep into the iridotomy site until perforation is obtained. The iridotomy can be enlarged by chipping at the margins of the opening. Shorter duration burns also will decrease bubble formation.

It is possible to destroy the pigment epithelium of blue irides by using excessively high power settings, thus leaving the stroma translucent but imperforate. Further treatment of such a site is futile because there will be inadequate pigment to absorb the laser energy. The power settings and duration of the burn should be adjusted so that definite stromal changes occur with each application. Power settings should be judiciously lowered as the duration of the burn time is increased. Then the power can be increased to obtain the desired effect on the stromal tissue. Burns of 0.2 sec duration using approximately 800 mW of power often are useful in patients with blue irides. Perforation can be obtained by interrupting the treatment session when the laser begins to have little effect and completing the treatment 30 to 60 minutes later when loose pigment collects around the iridotomy site.

Epithelial burns are common, particularly in the presence of corneal edema. They usually resolve within a few days and are not clinically significant in the long term, so long as the central cornea is avoided.[21,22] However, attempts to continue laser treatment through these opacities are usually fruitless and may lead to nonperforation. One can attempt to rotate the opacity out of the axis of treatment by changing the gaze position of the patient. Epithelial burns can be minimized by the reduction of corneal edema before laser therapy using ocular hypotensive drugs, osmotic agents, and topical glycerine. Second, the Abraham iridotomy lens will increase the cone angle of the beam and lessen the tissue effect at the corneal level. The lubricant between the lens and the cornea also will act as a heat sink to prevent coagulation of epithelial cells. The Abraham lens has a 66 D convex button that decreases the power density of the cornea fourfold by increasing the cone angle of the incident beam.[22] Corneal arcus should be avoided, since the opacified cornea is more likely to absorb energy and will create corneal burns and prevent perforation of the iris.

Endothelial burns occur more commonly than epithelial burns when the cornea is clear. They appear as white mucoid plaques and usually resolve within a week. They can prevent penetration of the iris by decreasing the power density at the level of the treatment site. Again, the convergent beam of the Abraham lens helps reduce the incidence and severity of endothelial burns by lessening the power density at the corneal level. If endothelial changes start to appear, the power or duration of the laser burns should be reduced, and the laser beam should be angled around the area of opacity.[23]

Occasionally, epithelial or endothelial burns preclude successful iridotomy.[24] The pupillary block may then be temporarily broken by peaking the pupil with one or more radial strings of contiguous burns using moderately large spot size and low power settings (200 μm, 200–300 mW, and 0.1–0.2 secs) (Fig. 18–7). Each string begins at the pupillary margin and extends as far

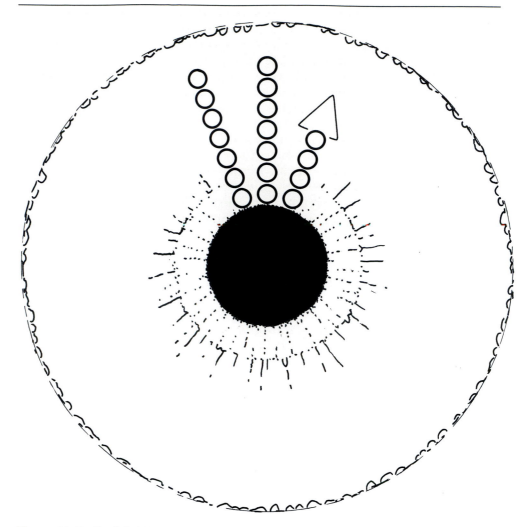

Figure 18–7. Radial strings of contiguous laser burns are used to peak the pupil and temporarily break the pupillary block; 200 μm, 200 to 300 mW, and 0.1 are typical settings.

peripherally as possible. Usually three to five adjacent strings are required before deepening of the anterior chamber is seen. This procedure will relieve the block for days to weeks, allowing an iridotomy to be completed when the chamber stabilizes.

After perforation is achieved, several postoperative complications may be encountered. First, the patient may complain of monocular diplopia. This potential problem can be avoided by choosing an iridotomy site covered by the upper lid, and in proximity to the 12-o'clock position.

Anterior subcapsular lenticular opacities commonly are seen posterior to the iridotomy. These cataractous changes are nonprogressive and only of visual significance if the iridotomy is placed near the visual axis. Asymptomatic peripheral retinal burns have been noted after laser iridotomy.[21] The chance of a visually destructive retinal burn can be reduced by choosing a peripheral site for the iridotomy, by focusing sharply on the iris, by angulating away from the fovea, and by using the Abraham lens, which increases the divergence of the laser beam behind the iris, thus reducing the power density at the level of the retina by approximately 17 times.

After a successful iridotomy, intraocular pressure may rise as high as 50 mm Hg. It usually returns to normal within hours. Eyes with compromised optic nerves deserve close observation postoperatively and may require additional hypotensive medication.

A transient nongranulomatous anterior uveitis frequently follows laser iridotomy. This complication usually resolves within a week. Rarely, a more severe protracted granulomatous or nongranulomatous response may require topical corticosteroid therapy and mydriatic agents.[22]

At least 5 percent of initially patent iridotomies close.[21,22] At the time of initial treatment, the incidence of closure can be minimized by carefully clearing the iridotomy of all bridging stromal strands. Unless the glaucoma is uveitic or rubeotic in nature, closure usually occurs within the first 6 postoperative weeks. Frequent observations should continue over this period as miotics are judiciously withdrawn. Occlusion is due to proliferation of pigment epithelium over the iridotomy side, and secondary opening is achieved easily with a minimum number of burns.

TRABECULOPLASTY

Trabeculoplasty is performed by using 50 μm spot size, 0.1 sec duration, and sufficient power to attain blanching of the trabecular meshwork with minimal vaporization (about 700–1200 mW). Eyes usually are treated in divided sessions, placing 50 burns over 180 degrees of the trabecular meshwork.[25–27]

Numerous high-intensity burns can induce open-angle glaucoma in animals.[28] As few as one hundred burns over 180 degrees can induce extensive angle closure through peripheral anterior synechia formation in a human eye. Retreatment over previously treated areas has yielded variable results, although the success rate is relatively low.[26,29] For these reasons, the accepted protocol should be altered significantly, and retreatment should be reserved for patients who are poor candidates for filtration surgery.

Treatment causes small hemorrhages in less than 5 percent of eyes.[26,30] Bleeding may arise from the burn or from adjacent tissues. It usually starts during treatment, although hemorrhaging has been observed during gonioscopy 5 weeks after laser surgery.[26] Occasionally, intraoperative bleeding will obscure the meshwork, and the laser session will have to be stopped. Fortunately, these minidiatheses usually stop spontaneously. Bleeding may be minimized by pushing on the contact lens to raise intraocular pressure or by photocoagulation of the source with 200 μm spots, 250 mW, 0.2 sec duration. The blood clears from the anterior chamber rapidly without affecting the intraocular pressure.

When given according to protocol, trabeculoplasty causes peripheral anterior synechiae in 29 to 47 percent of eyes. These synechiae are scattered and do not lead to creeping angle closure and do not affect the success rate of laser surgery.[25,28]

Mild uveitis frequently follows argon laser trabeculoplasty. The degree of uveitis has no effect on intraocular pressure, and it resolves rapidly. Those who use corticosteroids usually prescribe prednisolone acetate 1 percent or a similar drug four times daily or less for approximately 1 week.[25,26,31]

Corneal epithelial opacities have been noted after laser trabeculoplasty, but these clear within a few days. Corneal endothelial burns are very uncommon and rarely lead to permanent corneal decompensation. However, edema may last for several weeks in eyes with underlying corneal disease.[31]

Elevated intraocular pressure may develop in eyes after laser trabeculoplasty. For this reason the intraocular pressure can be checked every hour for 3 hours after laser trabeculoplasty. If the pressure peak falls within an acceptable range, the patient is checked again in 5 to 7 days and, if the pressure is satisfactory, rechecked 1 month postoperatively. In a minority of eyes (about 6 percent), the pressure reaches levels that threaten the optic nerve in the first 3 hours after laser treatment, and medical intervention is instituted. Treatment usually consists of oral glycerol (1.5 to 3.0 mL/kg of a 50 percent solution) because these patients are already on maximum tolerated medical therapy. Close observation is continued until the pressure falls sufficiently to protect the optic nerve. The patient may require daily visits until the pressure stabilizes at a tolerable level, and surgical intervention rarely is required to control postlaser pressure spikes. The use of iopidine and cold compresses in the immediate postlaser period may reduce the incidence of significant postlaser pressure elevation.

By dividing the trabeculoplasty into two sessions, the peak pressure elevation can be decreased significantly. It is unclear if divided sessions will prevent those rare pressure spikes that produce visual jeopardy.[32]

The pressure-lowering effect of trabeculoplasty may not be noted for 3 to 4 weeks. In a small number of eyes, a permanent rise in intraocular pressure follows trabeculoplasty. If there is inadequate intraocular pressure control, timely intervention with another surgical technique is indicated.

REFERENCES

1. Boulton PE, Brown N, Hamilton AM, Cheng H, Blach RK: A study of the mechanisms of transient myopia following extensive xenon arc photocoagulation. *Trans Ophthalmol Soc UK* 1973;93:287–300.
2. Huamonte FU, Peyman GA, Goldberg MF, Locketz A: Immediate fundus complications after retinal scatter photocoagulation: I. Clinical picture and pathogenesis. *Ophthalmic Surg* 1976;7:88–99.
3. Blondeau P, Pavan PR, Phelps CD: Acute pressure elevation following panretinal photocoagulation. *Arch Ophthalmol* 1981;99:1239–1241.
4. Doft BH, Blankenship GW: Single versus multiple treatment sessions of argon laser panretinal photocoagulation for proliferative diabetic retinopathy. *Ophthalmology* 1982;89:772–779.
5. Pavan PR, Ossoinig KC, Folk JC, Keen S: Incidence, type, and prognosis of neurosensory detachments following penretinal photocoagulation. *Invest Ophthalmol Vis Sci* 1982;22(suppl):51.
6. Meyers SM: Macular edema after scatter laser photocoagulation for proliferative diabetic retinopathy. *Am J Ophthalmol* 1980;90:210–216.
7. Ferris III FL, Podgor MJ, Davis MD: The Diabetic Retinopathy Study Research Group: macular edema in diabetic retinopathy study patients: diabetic retinopathy study report number 12. *Ophthalmology* 1987;94:754–760.
8. Last RJ, ed. *Wolff's Anatomy of the Eye and Orbit*, 6th ed. Philadelphia: WB Saunders Co; 1968:309–310.
9. Rogell GD: Internal ophthalmoplegia after argon laser panretinal photocoagulation. *Arch Ophthalmol* 1979;97:904–905.
10. Rutnin U: Fundus appearance in normal eyes: I. The choroid. *Am J Ophthalmol* 1967; 64:821–839.
11. The Diabetic Retinopathy Study Research Group: Photocoagulation treatment of proliferative diabetic retinopathy: clinical application of diabetic retinopathy study (DRS) findings, DRS report number 8. *Ophthalmology* 1981;88:583–600.
12. Pender PM, Benson WE, Compton H, Cox GB: The effects of panretinal photocoagulation on dark adaptation in diabetics with proliferative retinopathy. *Ophthalmology* 1981;88:635–638.
13. Chandra SR, Bresnick GH, Davis MD, Miller SA, Myers F: Choroidovitreal neovascular ingrowth after photocoagulation for proliferative diabetic retinopathy. *Arch Ophthalmol* 1980;98:1593–1599.
14. Francois J, DeLaey JJ, Cambie E, Hanssens M, Victoria-Troncoso V: Neovascularization after argon laser photocoagulation of macular lesions. *Am J Ophthalmol* 1975;79:206–210.

15. Hayreh SS, Weingeist TA: Experimental occlusion of the central artery of the retina: IV. Retinal tolerance time to acute ischaemia. *Br J Ophthalmol* 1980;64:818–825.
16. Yannuzzi LA, Shakin JL: Krypton red laser photocoagulation of the ocular fundus. *Retina* 1982;2:1–14.
17. Pavan PR, Folk JC: Anterior neovascularization. *Int Ophthalmol Clin* 1984;24:61–70.
18. Varley MP, Frank E, Purnell EW: Subretinal neovascularization after focal argon laser for diabetic macular edema. *Ophthalmology* 1988;95:567–573.
19. Lewis H, Schachat AP, Haimann MH, Haller JA, Quinlan P, Von Fricken MA, Fine SL, Murphy RP: Choroidal neovascularization after laser photocoagulation for diabetic macular edema. *Ophthalmology* 1990;97:503–511.
20. Trempe CL, Mainster MA, Pomerantzeff O, Avila MP, Jalkh AE, Weiter JJ, McMeel JW and Schepens CL: Macular photocoagulation: optimal wavelength selection. *Ophthalmology* 1982;89:721–728.
21. Pollach IP: Use of argon laser energy to produce iridotomies. *Trans Am Ophthalmol Soc* 1979;77:674–706.
22. Abraham RK: Protocol for single session argon laser iridectomy for angle-closure glaucoma. *Int Ophthalmol Clin* 1981;21:145–166.
23. Mandelkorn RM, Mendelsohn AD, Olander KW, Zimmerman TJ: Short exposure times in argon laser iridotomy. *Ophthal Surg* 1981;12:805–809.
24. Podos SM, Kels BD, Moss AP, Ritch R, Anders MD: Continuous wave argon laser iridectomy in angle-closure glaucoma. *Am J Ophthalmol* 1979;88:836–842.
25. Schwartz AL, Whitten ME, Bleiman B, Martin D: Argon laser trabecular surgery in uncontrolled phakic open-angle glaucoma. *Ophthalmology* 1981;88:203–212.
26. Thomas JV, Simmons RJ, Belcher III CD: Argon laser trabeculoplasty in the presurgical glaucoma patient. *Ophthalmology* 1982;89:187–197.
27. Wise JB, Witter SL: Argon laser therapy for open-angle glaucoma: a pilot study. *Arch Ophthalmol* 1979;97:319–322.
28. Gaasterland D, Kupfer C: Experimental glaucoma in the rhesus monkey. *Invest Ophthalmol* 1974;13:455–457.
29. Forbes M, Bansal RK: Argon laser goniophotocoagulation of the trabecular meshwork in open-angle glaucoma. *Trans Am Ophthalmol Soc* 1981;79:257–275.
30. Wise JB: Long-term control of adult open-angle glaucoma by argon laser treatment. *Ophthalmology* 1981;88:197–202.
31. Wilensky JT, Jampol LM: Laser therapy for open-angle glaucoma. *Ophthalmology* 1981;88:213–217.
32. Weinreb RN, Ruderman J, Juster R, Wilensky JT: Influence of the number of laser burns administered on the early results of argon laser trabeculoplasty. *Am J Ophthalmol* 1983;95:287–292.

Index

Page numbers followed by *t* and *f* refer to tables and figures, respectively.

Branch retinal vein occlusion (BRVO) (cont.)
preretinal neovascularization of,
photocoagulation of, 69, 71, 73–74f, 74t
Bruch's membrane
anatomy of, 5–6
in grade III lesions, 21, 23, 24
in grade II lesions, 19
in grade I lesions, 18
rupture of, 55, 135, 136, 182, 189–190
Bubble formation, in argon laser iridotomy, 195
Burn lesions
grade I, 18–19f
acute stage of, 17f, 18
chronic stage of, 18, 19f
clinical significance of, 18–19
grade II
acute stage of, 17f, 19
in chronic stage, 19–20f
clinical significance of, 20–21
grade III, 21, 22f
mild, 21–22, 23f
moderate, 23–24f
severe, 25–26f

C

Canal of Schlemm, 2f
Cantholysis, 191f
Carboxymethylcellulose sodium, 8
Central serous retinopathy
diagnosis of, 77
guidelines for photocoagulation, 78t
indications for treatment, 77–78
photocoagulation of, 78–80f
severe forms of, 80
Chamber angle, anatomy of, 1–2f
Choriocapillaris, 6
Chorioid, anatomy of, 5–6
Choroidal hemangioma
diagnosis of, 122–123
laser treatment, 124f–126f
alternatives, 123
complications, 123–124
follow-up, 123–124
techniques, 123, 124t
wavelength selection, 123
Choroidal neovascular membrane
in aging macular degeneration, signs of,
90–93f
drusen and, 85
in idiopathic juxtafoveal retinal telangiectasis,
116t, 117
in the presumed ocular histoplasmosis syndrome, 93–94
treatment of, 95t
Ciliary body, 1–2f
Closure of iridotomy, 145
Coagulation, of eye tissue, 1
Coats' syndrome. See Primary retinal
telangiectasis

Collector channels, 2
Complications of laser photocoagulation,
185–198
Contact lenses. See also Goldmann lenses
anterior segment lenses, 9
antireflection coatings of, 8
contraindications for laser surgery, 8–9
coupling solutions for, 8
Hoskins nylon suture laser lens, 9
Krieger, 10, 11t
Landers, 176
for laser surgery, features of, 8
Mainster, 11t, 12f, 48
ophthalmoscopic laser, 11t
posterior segment lenses, 9–13f
Ritch, 150
Rodenstock, 8, 11t
Volk, 12, 134
Wise, 9, 141
Yanuzzi, 10, 50
Contact lens solutions, 8
Corneal edema, 140–141
Corneal opacities
after binocular indirect ophthalmoscope laser
photocoagulation, 182
after iridotomy, 145
after trabeculoplasty, 155
Coupling solutions, 8
Cryopexy
for choroidal hemangioma, 123
for primary retinal telangiectasis, 114–115
for retinal angiomas, 109
for retinal breaks, 131
Cyclocryotherapy, 159–160
Cyclodiathermy, 159
Cyclophotocoagulation
endophotocoagulation, 161–162t
historical aspects of, 159–160
transpupillary, 160–161t
transscleral YAG
contact, 164–165t
noncontact, 163–164t
Cytomegalovirus, retinal breaks and, 130

D

Diabetic macular edema
diagnosis of, 57–58
diffuse, laser photocoagulation of, 61–65f
fluorescein angiography of, 57
focal
diagnosis of, 57
laser photocoagulation of, 58t, 59–61f
laser treatment, preferred laser wavelength
for, 58–59
Diabetic retinopathy, proliferative
contraction stage of, 31
diagnosis, prelaser examination, 45–46
and edematous retina with background
changes, 54
with extramacular tractional retinal detachment, 54f, 55f
florid diabetic retinopathy subgroup, 31–32f
follow-up, 52–53
krypton red laser for, 54–55

Page numbers followed by t and f refer to tables and figures, respectively.

Page numbers followed by *t* and *f* refer to tables and figures, respectively.

Page numbers followed by *t* and *f* refer to tables and figures, respectively.